KETO Simple

OVER 100 DELICIOUS LOW-CARB MEALS THAT ARE EASY ON TIME, BUDGET, AND EFFORT

FAIR WINDS

Martina Slajerova

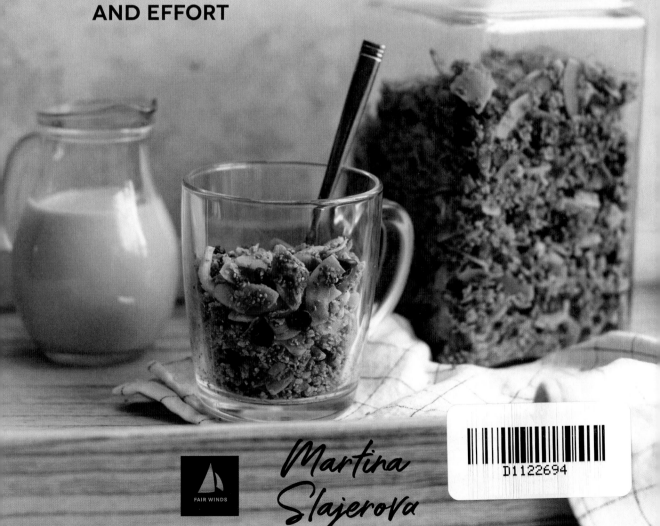

Brimming with creative inspiration, how-to projects, and useful information to enrich your everyday life, Quarto Knows is a favorite destination for those pursuing their interests and passions. Visit our site and dig deeper with our books into your area of interest: Quarto Creates, Quarto Cooks, Quarto Homes, Quarto Lives, Quarto Drives, Quarto Explores, Quarto Gifts, or Quarto Kids.

First Published in 2020 by Fair Winds Press, an imprint of The Quarto Group,
100 Cummings Center, Suite 265-D, Beverly, MA 01915, USA.
T (978) 282-9590 F (978) 283-2742 QuartoKnows.com

Fair Winds Press titles are also available at discount for retail, wholesale, promotional, and bulk purchase. For details, contact the Special Sales Manager by email at specialsales@quarto.com or by mail at The Quarto Group, Attn: Special Sales Manager, 100 Cummings Center, Suite 265-D, Beverly, MA 01915, USA.

23 22 21 20 19   1 2 3 4 5

ISBN: 978-1-59233-932-7

Digital edition published in 2020
eISBN: 978-1-63159-837-1

Library of Congress Cataloging-in-Publication Data is available.
Library of Congress Control Number: 2019954275

Design: Quarto Publishing Group USA
Cover Images: Martina Slajerova and Gwyn Cole (back cover, center)
Photography: Martina Slajerova and Gwyn Cole (page 5)

Printed in Canada

The information in this book is for educational purposes only. It is not intended to replace the advice of a physician or medical practitioner. Please see your health-care provider before beginning any new health program.

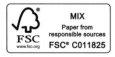

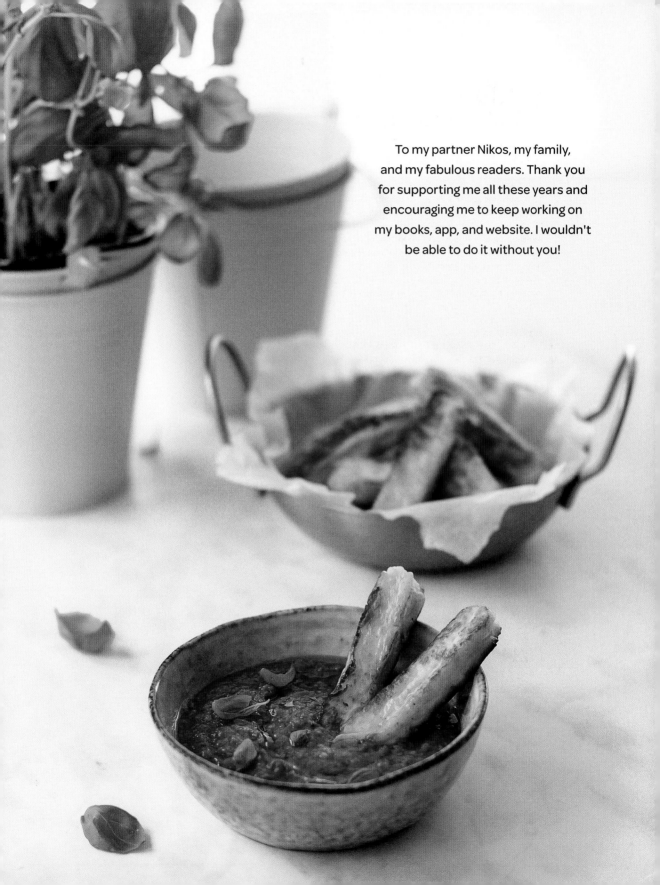

To my partner Nikos, my family, and my fabulous readers. Thank you for supporting me all these years and encouraging me to keep working on my books, app, and website. I wouldn't be able to do it without you!

Contents

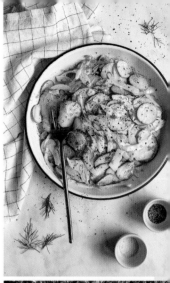

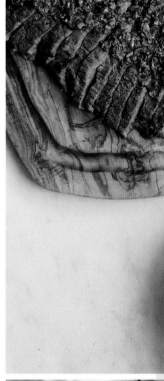

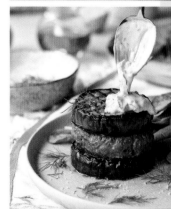

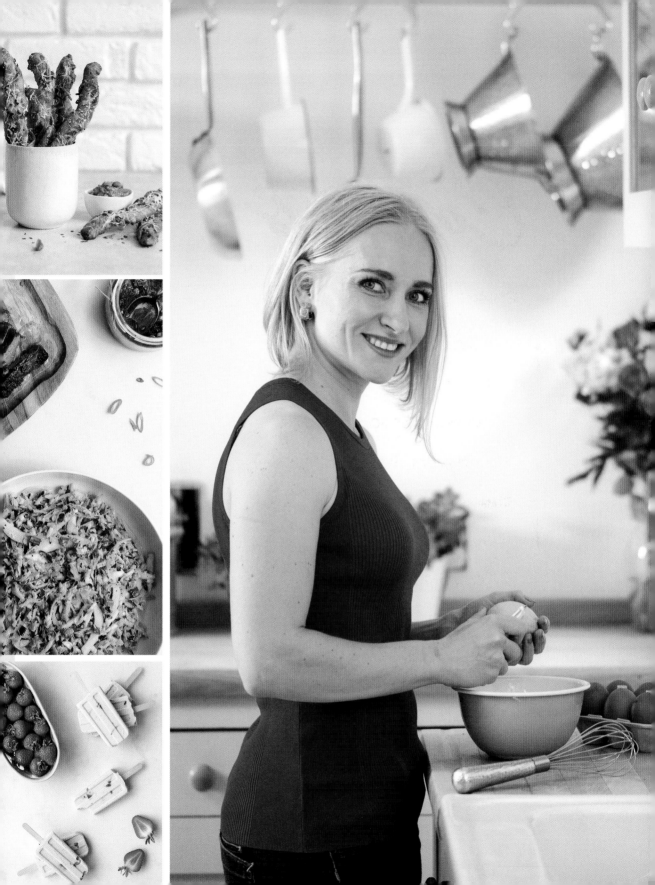

Chapter 1

Why Simle Keto?

None of us want to spend life endlessly thinking about the next meal. Counting calories is exhausting and it never works in the long term. Dieting becomes a burden instead of a tool to help us get healthier. We lose focus on things that really matter to us, and diets end up dictating how to live our lives. That's not just wrong—it's unsustainable.

The truth is that calorie-restricted diets are only short-term fixes and they are impossible to follow in the long term. The solution to this madness is simple: Find a way to eat to live—not the other way around.

What Is Keto?

In simple terms, when you follow a keto diet—low in carbs, moderate in protein, and high in fat—your blood sugar and insulin levels will stabilize. As a result, you will feel less hungry and naturally eat less. That's why low-carb eating is unlike any other dietary approach. On a keto diet, your body switches from glucose to fat as fuel, and you essentially become a fat burner. The main advantage of following a keto diet is that there is no calorie counting. Dieters can eat to satiety and easily maintain a healthy weight.

A low-carb diet is the first step toward a healthier you—but it's not the ultimate fix. I'm no stranger to "dieting" and I know that healthy eating can be really challenging. We've all been there: You start following a low-carb diet. You feel great and motivated. You lose weight. But you soon reach a weight loss plateau and suddenly your low-carb eating feels too overwhelming. You fail, and you are back to square one.

That's why it's time to change the way you think about low-carb eating. What's my secret? Keeping my diet simple. For me, low-carb is not a diet, it's a lifestyle. I have followed a healthy low-carb diet since 2011 and I don't even think about it anymore because **that's just the way I eat.**

But What If My Diet Is Not "Perfect"?

One of the most challenging parts about healthy eating is that it seems too complicated or too time-consuming—or both. We spend too much time trying to figure out how to make our diet perfect. The truth is that no matter what dietary approach you follow, it won't work if you strive for perfection.

The answer is KEEP IT SIMPLE. What does it mean? **Following keto is about more than just counting macros. It's about adopting a healthier lifestyle.**

Focus on your main goal (e.g., I want to stabilize my blood sugar, lose weight, etc.) and don't beat yourself up for details such as when you went a bit over your daily carb limit. Instead of punishing yourself, reward yourself for the positive steps you've taken, learn from your mistakes, and use them to your benefit.

There is no one dietary approach that fits all. Different activity levels, health conditions, gender, age, and lifestyle all play a significant role. Simply put, you have to find what works best for you and your specific needs. I hope my book will help you on your keto journey.

Simple Keto 101

Here's a quick guide to keto-friendly foods that'll help you make the right choices. (To find a comprehensive ketogenic food list, check out my blog: ketodietapp.com/blog.)

What to Eat

Eggs. Look for organic eggs, eggs from pastured chickens, and duck eggs.

Meat. Opt for grass-fed, humanely raised meat. When shopping on a budget, opt for antibiotic- and hormone-free sources, buy meat in bulk, and buy locally. Organ meats are an excellent source of protein, vitamins, and minerals. Be sure to watch out for hidden carbs in processed meats.

Wild-caught fish and organic farmed fish. You can find your best choices at seafoodwatch.org.

Dairy. Full-fat yogurt, hard cheese, soft cheese, cream, and butter are healthy options for those who can tolerate dairy.

Oils and fats. Look for pastured lard, grass-fed beef tallow, chicken fat, duck fat, goose fat, ghee, butter, virgin coconut oil, and sustainably sourced palm kernel oil. Butter is ideal for finishing meals or for light cooking. Extra-virgin olive oil, avocado oil, almond oil, and maca-damia oil are best for cold use, stir-fries, finishing meals, or after cooking. Nut and seed oils such as walnut, hazelnut, flaxseed, sesame seed, and pumpkin seed oil are only suitable for cold use.

Nuts and seeds. Include some of these in your diet: macadamia nuts, pecans, almonds, walnuts, hazelnuts, pine nuts, Brazil nuts, flaxseed, pumpkin seeds, sesame seeds, sunflower seeds, and hemp seeds. Nut and seed butters, coconut, and cacao butter are also good choices. Beware of cashew nuts and pistachios; they're relatively high in carbs.

Dark, leafy greens. Include a variety of greens in your diet, such as spinach, arugula, watercress, Swiss chard, kale, collards, bok choy, lettuce, and beet greens.

Low-carb vegetables. Choose cabbage, cauliflower, Brussels sprouts, zucchini, broccoli, tomatoes, peppers, radishes, daikon, okra, turnips, rutabaga, cucumber, celery, eggplant, asparagus, pumpkin, spaghetti squash, kohlrabi, sea vegetables, and mushrooms.

Low-carb fruits. Keto-friendly fruits include raspberries, blackberries, strawberries, blueberries, blackcurrants, lemon, lime, rhubarb, coconut, and avocado.

Minimally processed fermented soy products. Tempeh, natto, and tamari can be included.

Foods to Use Wisely

Fresh or dried herbs and spices can add so much to a simple dish. Just be sure to watch out for added sugar and starches in spice blends. When choosing condiments, look for unsweetened products with recognizable ingredients and minimal processing. To satisfy your sweet tooth, there are lots of healthy low-carb sweeteners (see conversion chart on page 12). Dark chocolate (minimum of 85% cacao content), raw cacao powder, and unsweetened 100% chocolate or sugar-free chocolate sweetened with stevia, monk fruit, or erythritol are also good options. Look for quality protein powder (additive- and sugar-free, no more than 5 grams of carbs per 100 grams), gelatin powder, and collagen powder. And don't forget that there are plenty of keto-friendly baking ingredients available.

Foods to Avoid

All grains, products made from grains, and potatoes. This includes wheat, rye, oats, corn, barley, millet, bulgur, sorghum, rice, amaranth, buckwheat, sprouted grain, quinoa, pasta, bread, pizza, cookies, crackers, etc.

All foods high in carbs and sugar. This includes cakes, cookies, ice cream, agave syrup, honey, tropical fruit and most high-sugar fruit, dried fruit, cocktails, sugary soft drinks, beer, etc.

All processed, inflammatory fats. This includes margarine, vegetable oil, soybean oil, etc.

Processed products containing soy. This is especially important if you suffer from hormone disorders.

Products labeled "low-fat" and "low-carb." These often contain hidden carbs and other unwanted ingredients.

Factory-farmed pork and non-organic farmed fish.

Alcohol, except low-carb options. Alcohol should be avoided for weight loss, as it stimulates appetite and is high in calories.

Carbohydrates on a Keto Diet

When following a ketogenic diet, aim for no more than 50 grams of total carbohydrates (20 to 30 grams of net carbohydrates) per day, mostly from non-starchy vegetables, avocados, and nuts. Everyone tolerates a slightly different carbohydrate level, and you'll need to find out what works best for you. Cutting all carbs from your diet is unnecessary and won't lead to an enhanced fat loss.

Don't obsess over your ketone levels. Ketone levels will show you how much "fuel" you have in your "tank," but not how much fuel your body is using for energy. Keto-adapted individuals are more likely to have lower ketone levels, simply because their bodies can use them more effectively than non-keto-adapted individuals.

Protein on a Keto Diet

When following a keto diet, keep your protein moderate at 0.6 to 1 gram per pound (1.3 to 2.2 grams per kilogram) of lean mass. In most cases, this translates to 65 to 80 grams of protein per day, sometimes even more. The exact amount depends on gender, lean mass weight, and activity level. Make sure you are eating enough and don't worry if you go over your protein intake. Eating slightly more protein will not slow down weight loss. Remember, protein is the most sating macronutrient; it will help you feel less hungry and eat fewer calories.

If your weight loss stalls on a keto diet, consuming too little fat probably isn't the cause. Try eating a bit more protein, as it provides appetite suppression, increases metabolic rate, and helps preserve muscle mass.

The fear some keto dieters have is that high protein intake leads to gluconeogenesis, a process by which the liver makes glucose from amino acids and other compounds. In most cases, protein is a self-limiting nutrient, meaning it is difficult to overeat, at least on a regular basis. Note: If you are insulin resistant or diabetic, or if you are managing a health condition, be aware that not all protein sources are equal. Consult your doctor.

Fat on a Keto Diet

When following a ketogenic diet, use fat as a "filler" to sate your appetite while keeping carbs low. Note that you likely won't need to watch your fat intake and count calories, but it may help as you reach a plateau especially when you get close to your target weight. If you want to find your ideal calorie intake, check out the KetoDiet App at ketodietapp.com. Apart from tracking carbs, protein, fat, and electrolytes, the app includes thousands of low-carb recipes to inspire your keto living!

The Importance of Electrolytes

During the initial phase of the ketogenic diet, you may experience headaches, nausea, fatigue, brain fog, muscle weakness, cramps, and heart palpitations. Don't panic. "Keto flu" is a natural process. I've experienced most of the symptoms myself, and if you're not prepared for it, these symptoms may scare you.

To minimize or even avoid the symptoms of keto flu, eat plenty of electrolyte-rich foods such as avocados, salmon, and spinach. Be sure to stay hydrated. Use salt and include magnesium supplements if needed. (Note: Consult your doctor before taking magnesium supplements if you have kidney disease or take medications for high blood pressure.) If you exercise, you may feel tired, so don't push yourself too much.

Simple Keto Hacks to Save Time & Money

The reason I've been able to follow a low-carb diet for almost a decade is that I keep it as simple and practical as possible. Here are some of the strategies that work for me:

Prep your meals. Reserve time every week to prepare pantry basics (see page 14). It is totally worth it! Or go one step further and prepare all your meals on one day and then refrigerate or freeze for later.

Plan your meals. To keep planning easy, stick with recipes that require fewer ingredients and less hands-on time. That is what I focused on when creating recipes for this book!

Make a list. A shopping list is a must. It will save you time and money. Also, don't go shopping when you're hungry. I order most of my groceries online and find that it's easier to focus on what I really need.

Cook in bulk. No time to cook? Most recipes in this book take less than thirty minutes to prepare. Plus, they are easy to scale up. Choose two to three simple meals and double or triple the batch to have enough for the whole week!

Embrace variety. Make simple changes in recipes to a create a whole new meal. Swap the herbs and spices for other aromatics. Or change the protein and use different low-carb veggies. It's easy!

Stock up on essentials. To make cooking easy, stock up on frozen vegetables and berries, pantry essentials, condiments, canned fatty fish, nuts, and seeds.

Say yes to the helpful tools. Use a microwave, pressure cooker, or slow cooker to cut down your cooking time. I make an amazing chicken stock in my electric pressure cooker every week.

Get creative with your leftovers. Turn the meat from last night's dinner into tomorrow's lunch. Use wonky veg and mushrooms to make a simple frittata (page 24). Leftover herbs and even leafy greens are perfect for making Simple Pesto (page 16). Use leftover egg yolks to make hollandaise sauce, Creamy Breakfast Hot Chocolate (page 45) or Long-Lasting Mayonnaise (page 16).

Dining Out

Dining out on a ketogenic diet is much easier than you might think. Here are a few strategies to set you up for success:

Prepare ahead of time. Many restaurants share their menus online. If the menu isn't available in advance, ask for a gluten-free menu and look for the best keto options.

Avoid all high-carb foods and watch out for foods with hidden carbs. Choose dishes that are prepared simply, without sauces. Opt for grilled, baked, steamed, or roasted meats, poultry, seafood, non-starchy vegetables, or salads.

Double your order of non-starchy veg sides. Ask for keto salad dressing or for extra-virgin olive oil, lemon wedges, and vinegar (go easy on balsamic, as it's relatively high in carbs).

Still or carbonated water is always a safe choice, as is coffee or tea. Fresh-squeezed lemon or lime can jazz up water or club soda. Opt for distilled spirits, dry wine, and low-carb cider and beer (gluten-free options are available).

Finally, don't obsess over every detail. Just focus on your priorities—and enjoy yourself! For comprehensive guides to dining out on keto, visit my blog at ketodietapp.com/blog.

Simple Low-Carb Swaps

Pasta **>** zucchini noodles, shirataki noodles, or kelp noodles

Rice **>** cauli-rice (page 14) or shirataki rice

Roasted potatoes **>** chopped rutabaga, turnips, radishes, or cauliflower

Potato mash **>** cauliflower mash (page 66)

Soy sauce **>** coconut aminos or tamari sauce

Milk **>** unsweetened almond milk or coconut milk

Rice, bulgur, and quinoa **>** cauli-rice (page 14) or hulled hemp seeds

Crackers **>** Cheese Crisps (page 54), flaxseed crackers, celery sticks, cucumber slices, radishes, or sliced bell peppers; dehydrated vegetables; and beef jerky

Bread **>** Three-Minute Keto Bread (page 67); lettuce leaves to replace burger buns (page 124)

Tortillas **>** lettuce or chard leaves

Pizza **>** protein pizza crust (page 116)

Oats and cereals **>** chia seeds, unsweetened almonds, coconut flakes, hulled hemp seeds

High-carb alcoholic beverages (cocktails, beer, mixers) **>** dry martini, spirits, club soda, dry white and red wines, prosecco, champagne, low-carb cider and beer (gluten-free options are available).

You'll also find several other keto-friendly recipes, including bread, tortillas, crackers, and more, on my blog at ketodietapp.com/blog.

Sweetener Swaps

1 teaspoon sugar = 2 to 3 drops liquid stevia or monk fruit OR a pinch of pure powdered stevia or monk fruit OR 1 teaspoon erythritol or Swerve

1 tablespoon (10 g/0.4 oz) sugar = 6 to 9 drops liquid stevia or monk fruit OR ¼ teaspoon pure powdered stevia or monk fruit OR 1 tablespoon erythritol or Swerve

1 cup (200 g/7.1 oz) table (granulated) sugar = 1 cup (200 g/7.1 oz) granulated Swerve OR 1⅓ cups (267 g/9.4 oz) granulated erythritol OR 1 cup (200 g/7.1 oz) granulated stevia or monk fruit blend OR 1 teaspoon pure powdered stevia or monk fruit OR 1 teaspoon liquid stevia or liquid monk fruit

1 cup (160 g/5.6 oz) confectioners' sugar = 1 cup (160 g/5.6 oz) confectioners' Swerve OR 1⅓ cups (213 g/17.5 oz) confectioners' (powdered) erythritol

1 tablespoon (15 ml) honey, blackstrap molasses, or maple syrup = 2 tablespoons (30 ml) yacon syrup

Easy Substitutions When Cooking

1 clove fresh garlic = about ½ teaspoon minced garlic **>** ½ teaspoon garlic flakes, ¼ teaspoon granulated garlic, or ⅛ teaspoon garlic powder

1 small onion = about ⅓ cup (70 g/2.5 oz) chopped onion **>** 1 teaspoon onion powder or 1 tablespoon (5 g/0.2 oz) dried onion flakes

1 tablespoon (15 ml) lime juice **>** 1 tablespoon (15 ml) lemon juice or ½ tablespoon (8 ml) apple cider vinegar or wine vinegar

1 teaspoon baking powder **>** ½ teaspoon cream of tartar + ½ teaspoon baking soda OR ½ to 1 teaspoon lemon juice + ½ teaspoon baking soda

1 tablespoon (6 g/0.2 oz) fresh grated ginger/turmeric **>** ¼ teaspoon ginger powder/ turmeric powder

1 tablespoon fresh chopped herbs **>** 1 teaspoon dried herbs
Bone broth **>** beef stock, chicken stock, vegetable stock (same amounts)

How to Use This Book

NUTRITION FACTS

Nutrition values for each recipe in this book are per serving unless stated otherwise. The nutrition data are derived from the USDA National Nutrient Database (ndb.nal.usda.gov). Nutrition facts are calculated from edible parts. For example, if one large avocado is listed as 200 g/7.1 oz, this value represents its edible parts (pit and peel removed) unless otherwise specified. Optional ingredients and suggested sides and toppings are not included in the nutrition information. You can use raw cacao powder and unsweetened cocoa powder (Dutch-process) interchangeably. Ingredients are all full-fat unless otherwise specified. All ingredients should be sugar-free, unless you use dark 85% to 90% chocolate, which contains a small and acceptable amount of sugar.

All recipes are tagged with the following icons, as needed. These are the tags you will find in my recipes:

 dairy-free   nightshade-free

 nut-free   vegetarian

 egg-free   high in electrolytes

OPTIONAL INGREDIENTS

Optional ingredients, suggested sides, and suggested alternatives and toppings are not included in the nutrition information. If options are included, such recipes are tagged , etc. For example, Pesto Egg Drop Soup (page 78) calls for Simple Pesto (page 16) made with or without Parmesan, and therefore has the gray dairy-free icon .

AN IMPORTANT NOTE ABOUT MEASUREMENTS

It's better if you use a kitchen scale to measure ingredients; using cups or tablespoons can lead to inaccuracies and that may affect the recipe, especially when it comes to dry ingredients used in baked goods.

Keto Pantry Basics

Cauli-Rice
Shirataki Noodles • Fettucine • Rice
Bacon
Eggs
Long-Lasting Mayonnaise
Simple Pesto
Flavored Butter

Cauli-Rice

Wash the cauliflower and drain well. Once dry, grate with a hand grater or place the florets in a food processor with a grating blade and pulse until it looks like rice. Don't overdo it. It only takes a few more seconds to make purée out of your cauliflower. Place in a sealed container and store for up to 4 days.

Steaming: Place in a steam pot and cook for 5 to 7 minutes.

Microwaving: Place in a microwave-safe bowl and cook on medium-high for 5 to 7 minutes. No water needed.

Pan-roasting: You can briefly cook the cauli-rice in a pan greased with butter or ghee, or add it directly to the pot with meat or sauce you plan to serve it with. This method adds extra flavor to your cauli-rice!

Shirataki Noodles • Fettucine • Rice

Wash the shirataki noodles thoroughly. Boil them in a pot of water and a dash of apple cider vinegar for 2 to 3 minutes. Drain well. Place the noodles in a hot dry pan. Fry over medium-high heat for about 10 minutes. Using tongs, toss the noodles as they cook. Add the fried noodles directly to a meal, or place in a sealed container and refrigerate for up to 3 days.

Bacon

OVEN BAKING (BEST FOR LARGE AMOUNTS)

Preheat the oven to 320°F (160°C) forced fan or 355°F (180°C) conventional. Line a baking tray with parchment paper. Lay out the bacon in a single layer or lay on a wire rack set on top of the parchment. Cook in the oven for 25 to 30 minutes. Remove and let cool for 5 minutes. Strain the bacon grease into a small jar. Let the slices cool completely. Store in a sealed container in the fridge for up to 1 week or freeze for up to 3 months.

PAN-ROASTING (BEST FOR SMALLER AMOUNTS)

Place the bacon in a large pan and add ½ cup (120 ml) of water. Cook over medium-high heat until the water starts to boil. Reduce the heat to medium and cook until the water evaporates and the bacon fat is rendered. Reduce the heat to low and cook until the bacon is lightly browned and crispy. Let it cool slightly and cut it into pieces.

Eggs

BOILED EGGS

Fresh eggs don't peel well. Use eggs that you bought 7 to 10 days before cooking. Place the eggs in a pot and fill with water, covering them by an inch (2.5 cm). Bring to a boil over high heat. Turn off the heat and cover with a lid. Remove from the burner and keep the eggs covered in the pot (10 to 12 minutes for medium-size eggs; 13 to 14 minutes for large; 15 to 16 minutes for extra-large; 17 to 18 minutes for jumbo and duck eggs). When done, transfer to a bowl filled with ice water and let the eggs sit for 5 minutes. Once cooled, store unpeeled in the fridge for up to 1 week. To get the eggs soft-boiled, leave them covered in hot water for 5 to 7 minutes.

POACHED EGGS

Fill a medium saucepan with water and a dash of vinegar. Bring to a boil over high heat. Crack each egg individually into a ramekin or a cup. Using a spoon, create a gentle whirlpool in the water; this will help the egg white wrap around the egg yolk. Slowly lower the egg into the water in the center of the whirlpool. Turn off the heat and cook for 3 to 4 minutes. Use a slotted spoon to remove the egg from the water and place it on a plate. Repeat for all remaining eggs. Once cool, place all the eggs in a sealed container filled with cold water and keep refrigerated for up to 5 days. To reheat the eggs, place them in a mug filled with hot tap water for a couple of minutes. This will be enough to warm them up without overcooking.

PICKLED EGGS

Place peeled hard-boiled eggs into a jar filled with pickling liquid and let them marinate for at least 2 hours before eating. For about 1 L of pickling liquid, you simply need 3 cups (710 ml) of filtered water and 1 cup (240 ml) of vinegar. You can add any herbs, spices, and salt to taste.

CHIA EGGS

Egg-free? To substitute for 1 large egg: Mix together 1 tablespoon (8 g/0.3 oz) ground chia seeds or 1 tablespoon (7 g/0.2 oz) ground flaxseed or 1 tablespoon (11 g/0.4 oz) gelatin powder with 3 tablespoons (45 ml) water. This swap has limited use, as it won't work for mayonnaise, hollandaise, etc., but it is useful as a binder in patties (page 102) and meatballs (page 103).

Long-Lasting Mayonnaise (makes about 2 cups/480 ml)

Use a wide-mouth Mason jar that barely fits the head of your immersion blender. This is vital for the recipe to work. Place 2 large egg yolks, 2 teaspoons Dijon mustard (or nightshade-free yellow mustard), 2 tablespoons (30 ml) apple cider vinegar, 2 tablespoons (30 ml) fresh lemon juice, ½ teaspoon fine sea salt, and ¼ teaspoon ground black pepper in the jar. Pour 1½ cups (360 ml) walnut oil (or macadamia, avocado, or light olive oil) on top, and let it settle for 20 seconds. Place the head of the immersion blender at the bottom of the jar and turn it on high speed. (Do not pulse.) As the mayonnaise thickens, gently tilt and move the head of the immersion blender until the mayonnaise is thick. Add 2 tablespoons (30 ml/1 oz) whey (the liquid part on top of raw full-fat yogurt) or powder from 1 to 2 probiotic capsules or non-dairy options such as sauerkraut juice or fermented pickle juice. Cover the jar loosely with a lid or a cloth, and let it sit on the kitchen counter for 8 hours. This is essential in order to activate the enzymes that will keep your mayo fresh. Refrigerate after 8 hours and use within the next 3 months.

Note: When using raw eggs, prevent any health risks by using eggs with pasteurized shells. To pasteurize eggs at home, simply pour enough water into a saucepan to cover the eggs. Heat to about 140°F (60°C). Using a spoon, slowly place the eggs in the saucepan. Keep the eggs in the water for about 3 minutes. This should be enough to pasteurize the eggs and kill any potential bacteria. Let cool, then store in the fridge for 6 to 8 weeks.

Simple Pesto (makes about 1 cup /240 ml)

Place all the ingredients in a blender: 2 cups (30 g/1.1 oz) fresh basil or herbs of choice (parsley, cilantro, and mint work best); ⅓ cup (45 g/1.6 oz) macadamia nuts, blanched almonds, or hulled sunflower seeds; 2 tablespoons (15 g/0.5 oz) pine nuts or more sunflower seeds; 4 cloves minced garlic; 1 teaspoon fresh lemon zest; 1 tablespoon (15 ml) fresh lemon juice; and ½ cup (120 ml) extra-virgin olive oil. Optionally, you can add ⅓ cup (30 g/1.1 oz) grated Parmesan cheese and/or 4 to 6 pieces of drained sun-dried tomatoes. Process until smooth, then season with sea salt and black pepper to taste.

You can keep your pesto in the fridge for up to 1 to 2 weeks. Always remember to add a thin layer of olive oil on top before you place it back in the fridge. Or spoon it into an ice cube tray and place in the freezer. Once frozen, empty the tray into a resealable plastic bag. Keep your frozen pesto for up to 6 months.

Flavored Butter (1 small log)

Combine 4 oz (115 g) room temperature butter with a pinch of salt and pepper and add 1 to 2 tablespoons of any fresh herbs (or 1 to 2 teaspoons dried herbs). You can also add other ingredients such as fresh lemon zest, spices (cumin, paprika, curry powder, etc.), crumbled bacon, or grated cheese. Keep the butter in a bowl stored in the fridge or shape it into a small log by wrapping it in a piece of parchment paper. Flavored butter can be refrigerated for up to 1 week or frozen for up to 6 months.

Note: For even more keto basics, including bone broth, nut and seed milk, activated nuts, ketchup, BBQ sauce, mustard, harissa paste, curry paste, chile paste, and more, visit ketodietapp.com/blog.

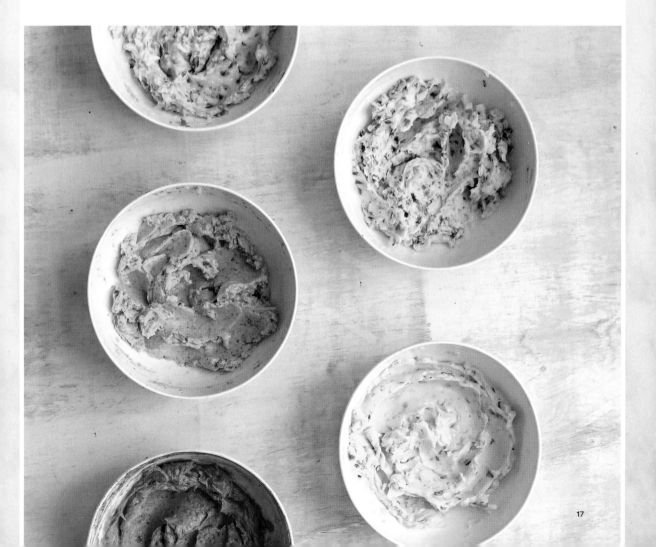

Chapter 2
Breakfasts

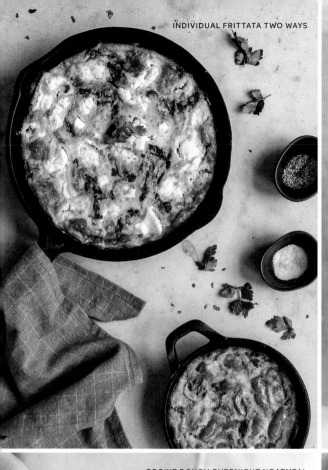

INDIVIDUAL FRITTATA TWO WAYS

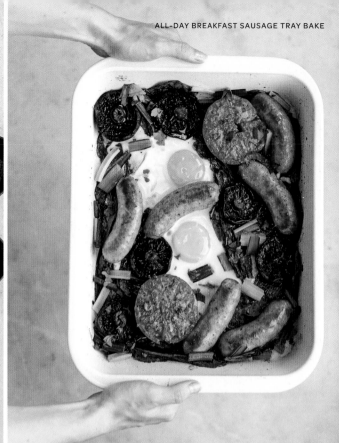

ALL-DAY BREAKFAST SAUSAGE TRAY BAKE

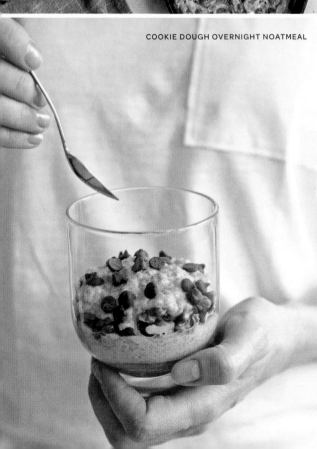

COOKIE DOUGH OVERNIGHT NOATMEAL

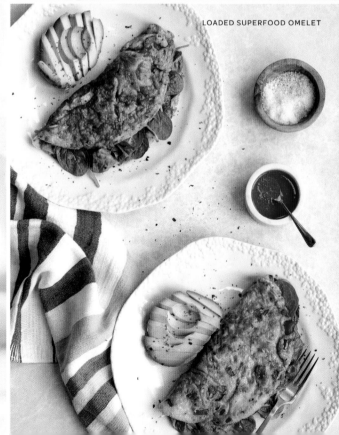

LOADED SUPERFOOD OMELET

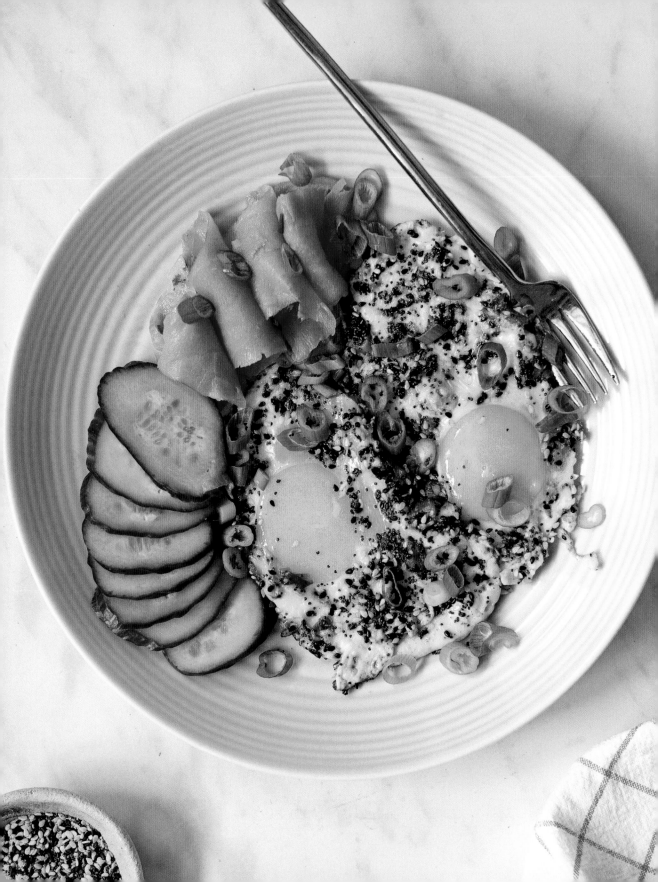

Everything Bagel Eggs

SERVINGS: 1
HANDS-ON TIME: 10 minutes
OVERALL TIME: 10 minutes

This simple recipe takes under 10 minutes and features your favorite bagel topping. The seasoning tastes great with fried eggs, sprinkled on salads, sliced avocado, or roasted veggies!

1 tablespoon (15 ml) ghee or duck fat

2 large eggs

1 tablespoon (14 g/0.5 oz) everything bagel seasoning (see tip for homemade)

½ small (57 g/2 oz) sliced cucumber

2 ounces (57 g) smoked salmon

1 medium (15 g/0.5 oz) spring onion, sliced

Heat a pan greased with ghee over medium-high heat. Crack in the eggs and cook until the whites start turning opaque. Sprinkle with the seasoning and cook until the whites are set and the yolk is still runny. Serve immediately with sliced cucumber, salmon, and spring onion.

TIP:

To make your own "everything bagel seasoning," simply mix:

    1 tablespoon (9 g/0.3 oz) white sesame seeds

    1 tablespoon (9 g/0.3 oz) black sesame seeds

    1½ tablespoons (13 g/0.5 oz) poppy seeds

    1 tablespoon (3 g/0.1 oz) dried minced onion (or 1 teaspoon onion powder)

    1 tablespoon (3 g/0.1 oz) dried minced garlic (or 1 teaspoon garlic powder)

    1 teaspoon flaked or coarse sea salt

This will yield about ¼ cup (42 g/1.5 oz) of seasoning.

NUTRITION FACTS PER SERVING:
Total carbs: 5.9 g / Fiber: 2 g / Net carbs: 3.9 g / Protein: 25 g / Fat: 30.5 g / Calories: 402 kcal
Macronutrient ratio: Calories from carbs (4%), protein (26%), fat (70%)

Spiced Skillet Eggs with Yogurt

SERVINGS: 2
HANDS-ON TIME: 15 minutes
OVERALL TIME: 20 minutes

These breakfast skillet eggs are like a cross between Turkish eggs and shakshuka with smoky paprika, nutritious veggies, and full-fat yogurt.

1 tablespoon (15 ml) ghee or extra-virgin olive oil

½ small (35 g/1.2 oz) yellow onion, sliced

1 clove garlic, minced

1 teaspoon smoked paprika

1 medium (120 g/4.2 oz) green pepper, sliced

½ cup (120 g/4.2 oz) canned tomatoes

4 ounces (113 g) fresh spinach (or frozen and thawed spinach with juices squeezed out)

4 large eggs

Salt and pepper, to taste

1 tablespoon (4 g/0.2 oz) chopped parsley and/or mint

Red pepper flakes, to taste

½ cup (125 g/4.5 oz) full-fat Greek yogurt

1 tablespoon (15 ml) extra-virgin olive oil

Heat a pan greased with ghee over medium-high heat. Add the onion and cook for 5 minutes. Add the garlic, smoked paprika, green pepper, and tomatoes. Mix and cook for 5 minutes. Add the spinach and cook for just a minute, until wilted. Season with salt and pepper to taste. Make 4 small wells and crack an egg into each. Cover with a lid and cook for a few minutes, until the whites are opaque and the yolks are still runny. Take off the heat and season with salt and pepper, fresh herbs, and red pepper flakes. Serve with yogurt drizzled with olive oil.

NUTRITION FACTS PER SERVING:
Total carbs: 12.7 g / Fiber: 4.2 g / Net carbs: 8.5 g / Protein: 21.3 g / Fat: 27.5 g / Calories: 378 kcal
Macronutrient ratio: Calories from carbs (9%), protein (23%), fat (68%)

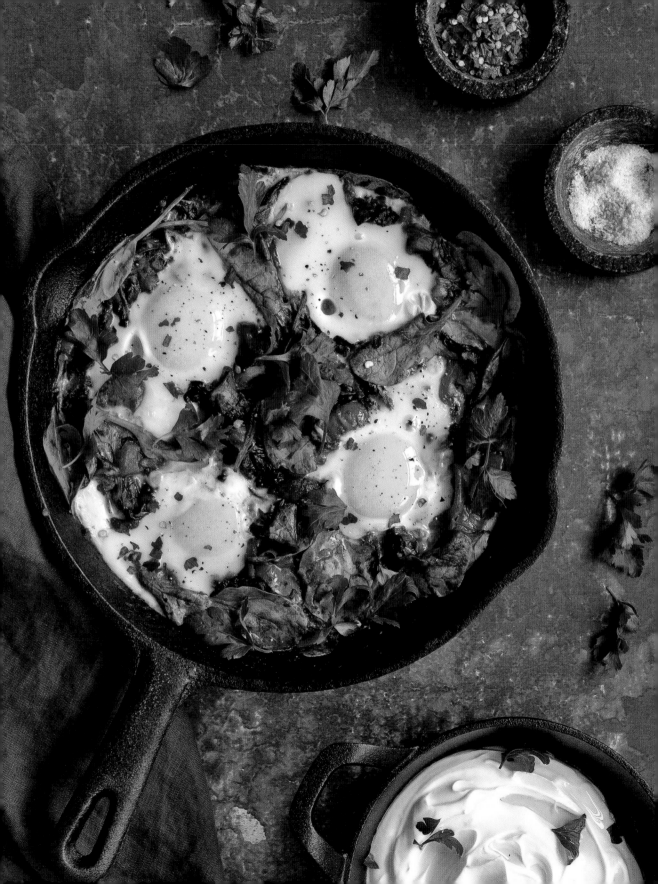

Individual Frittata Two Ways

SERVINGS: 1
HANDS-ON TIME: 10 minutes
OVERALL TIME: 20 minutes

There are endless ways to make a frittata. The base is simple, and the toppings can be adjusted to your liking. Cooking for the whole family? This recipe is really easy to scale up!

2 large eggs

1 tablespoon (15 ml) heavy whipping cream

1 tablespoon (5 g/0.2 oz) grated Parmesan cheese or any hard cheese

Pinch of salt and pepper

1 teaspoon ghee or duck fat

¼ small (20 g/0.7 oz) yellow onion, sliced

CHEESY SPINACH FRITTATA

2 cups (60 g/2.1 oz) fresh spinach (or frozen and thawed spinach with juices squeezed out)

2 ounces (57 g) soft goat's cheese or feta

CHORIZO & MUSHROOM FRITTATA

2 ounces (57 g) diced Spanish chorizo or bacon

3 pieces (57 g/2 oz) white mushrooms, sliced

In a bowl, lightly whisk the eggs, whipping cream, Parmesan cheese, salt, and pepper. Heat a small 6-inch (15 cm) skillet greased with ghee over medium-high heat (if you need to scale the recipe up, use a larger skillet). Add the onion and cook for a few minutes, until fragrant. Take off the heat.

FOR THE CHEESY SPINACH FRITTATA: Add the spinach and cook for about 30 seconds, until wilted. Pour in the egg-cream mixture and add chunks of goat's cheese. Take off the heat.

FOR THE CHORIZO & MUSHROOM FRITTATA: Add the chorizo and cook for 2 minutes, until the spicy juices are released. Add the mushrooms and cook for 3 to 5 minutes, until tender. Pour in the egg-cream mixture. Take off the heat.

FINAL STEPS: Place the frittata under a broiler for 3 to 5 minutes, until set and lightly browned. Serve immediately or let it cool and refrigerate for up to 4 days.

PICTURED ON PAGE 19

NUTRITION FACTS PER SERVING (CHEESY SPINACH/CHORIZO & MUSHROOM):
Total carbs: 5.2/6.1 g / Fiber: 1.8/1.3 g / Net carbs: 3.4/4.8 g / Protein: 27/30.4 g / Fat: 33.7/43.9 g
Calories: 434/546 kcal / Macronutrient ratio: Calories from carbs (3/4%), protein (25/23%), fat (72/73%)

Good-for-Your-Gut Bacon Hash

SERVINGS: 2
HANDS-ON TIME: 10 minutes
OVERALL TIME: 20 minutes

This six-ingredient breakfast hash is so versatile! I eat mine with sauerkraut and fried eggs, but you can add sliced avocado, crumbled feta, or grated Cheddar. Crisp it up under a broiler—yum!

8 slices (240 g/8.5 oz) bacon, chopped

1 cup (70 g/2.5 oz) sliced white mushrooms

8 leaves (120 g/4.2 oz) savoy cabbage, stems removed and sliced

1 tablespoon (18 g/0.7 oz) whole-grain mustard or Dijon mustard

2 large eggs, fried or poached

½ cup (47 g/1.7 oz) drained sauerkraut

Optional: salt, pepper, and red pepper flakes, to taste

Heat a large skillet over medium heat. Place the bacon in the skillet and add about ½ cup (120 ml) of water. Cook for 10 to 15 minutes, until the water evaporates and the bacon is crisp. Use a slotted spoon to transfer the bacon to a plate, leaving the rendered fat in the skillet.

To the skillet, add the mushrooms and cook for about 5 minutes. Add the cabbage and another ¼ cup (60 ml) of water. Stir to combine and cover with a lid. Cook for 5 minutes, then remove the lid and cook for another 2 minutes to allow the water to evaporate. Add the mustard and crisp bacon and cook briefly to heat through. Take off the heat and transfer to serving plates.

Top with the eggs and sauerkraut. Optionally, season with salt and pepper or red pepper flakes. The hash (without toppings) can be stored in the fridge for up to 4 days.

TIP:

Swap savoy cabbage for sliced Brussels sprouts, collards, spinach, or chard. If you're using tender greens such as chard or spinach, only cook the greens for 30 to 60 seconds. Swap the bacon for Mexican chorizo or gluten-free Italian sausage, plus add 2 tablespoons (30 ml) of ghee or duck fat. Swap the sauerkraut for fresh Mexican salsa or sliced avocado.

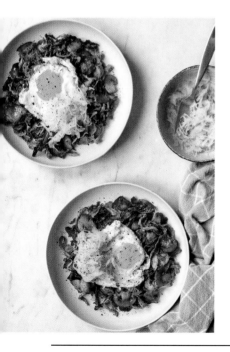

NUTRITION FACTS PER SERVING:
Total carbs: 7.5 g / Fiber: 3.5 g / Net carbs: 4 g / Protein: 26 g / Fat: 36.1 g / Calories: 454 kcal
Macronutrient ratio: Calories from carbs (4%), protein (23%), fat (73%)

Eggs Benedict with Avo-Feta Smash

SERVINGS: 1
HANDS-ON TIME: 10 minutes
OVERALL TIME: 10 minutes

This is a classic breakfast dish. Instead of bread rolls, this recipe uses our quick keto bread. I always keep some poached eggs in the fridge to make eggs benny in just a few minutes.

1 large egg, poached or fried

½ large (100 g/3.5 oz) avocado

2 teaspoons (10 ml) fresh lime or lemon juice

¼ cup (38 g/1.3 oz) crumbled feta cheese

Salt and pepper, to taste

2 ounces (57 g) sliced ham

1 piece Three-Minute Keto Bread (page 67)

Optional: fresh herbs of choice or microgreens

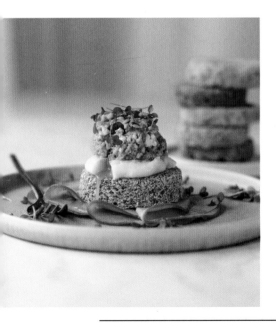

Start by cooking the egg (see page 15). Place the avocado and lime juice in a bowl, and smash with a fork. Add the feta and stir to combine. Season with salt and pepper.

TO ASSEMBLE THE DISH: Place the ham on a plate. Top with the keto bread, poached egg, and the avo-feta mixture. Optionally, sprinkle with fresh herbs or microgreens. Serve immediately.

TIPS:

• This meal is relatively high in fiber, which increases the total carb count. If you can't tolerate high-fiber meals, skip the bread and add an extra egg or serve with Baked Cauliflower Pancakes (page 38) or more avocado and feta topping. Instead of classic pork ham you can use smoked salmon, pastrami, Parma ham, or turkey ham.

• You can swap the avocado topping for Hollandaise sauce. To make two servings, heat 6 tablespoons (85 g/ 3 oz) of unsalted butter or ghee in a saucepan over medium heat until melted and bubbling. Take off the heat. Place 2 egg yolks in a blender with 1 tablespoon (15 ml) of fresh lemon juice, and a pinch of salt and pepper. Blend for a few seconds until the yolks are broken down. With the blender running, pour in the hot butter in a slow, steady stream until the mixture thickens. To thin down the sauce, optionally add a dash of water and blend again.

NUTRITION FACTS PER SERVING (USING BASIC THREE-MINUTE KETO BREAD):
Total carbs: 20.2 g / Fiber: 13.6 g / Net carbs: 6.6 g / Protein: 31.7 g / Fat: 44.2 g / Calories: 576 kcal
Macronutrient ratio: Calories from carbs (5%), protein (23%), fat (72%)

Loaded Superfood Omelet

SERVINGS: 1
HANDS-ON TIME: 10 minutes
OVERALL TIME: 10 minutes

Busy mornings don't have to mean eating the same boring meals! Omelets are a classic breakfast meal and this one is packed with flavor, vitamins, minerals, protein, and healthy fats.

1 tablespoon (15 ml) ghee or duck fat

¼ small (20 g/0.7 oz) yellow onion, sliced

3 large eggs

Pinch of salt and pepper

1 tablespoon (4 g/0.2 oz) chopped herbs of choice (parsley, cilantro, chives, or basil)

¼ cup (28 g/1 oz) shredded Cheddar or mozzarella cheese

¼ cup (28 g/1 oz) diced ham

½ medium (60 g/2.1 oz) red bell pepper, finely diced

1 cup (30 g/1.1 oz) fresh spinach (or frozen and thawed spinach with juices squeezed out)

Optional add-ons: ½ large (100 g/3.5 oz) sliced avocado, Sriracha sauce, and red pepper flakes

Heat a large skillet greased with ghee over medium heat. Add the onion and cook for 3 to 5 minutes, until fragrant.

In a small bowl, whisk the eggs with salt, pepper, and herbs. Pour the eggs into the pan and cook, lifting the edges with a spatula and tilting the pan to allow uncooked egg to run under the omelet.

When the omelet is almost cooked but still moist on top, add the cheese, ham, bell pepper, and spinach across the top of the omelet. Gently fold in half and cook for another 1 to 2 minutes, until cooked through. Eat immediately, topped with any optional add-ons you desire, or store in the fridge for up to 1 day.

PICTURED ON PAGE 19

NUTRITION FACTS PER SERVING:
Total carbs: 9 g / Fiber: 2.4 g / Net carbs: 6.6 g / Protein: 31.9 g / Fat: 40 g / Calories: 528 kcal
Macronutrient ratio: Calories from carbs (5%), protein (25%), fat (70%)

Kedgeree

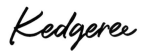

SERVINGS: 4
HANDS-ON TIME: 15 minutes
OVERALL TIME: 25 minutes

Traditional kedgeree is a hearty British-Indian meal that features smoked haddock, boiled eggs, and rice, and it is flavored with warming curry powder. In this recipe, we're using cauli-rice and adding nutrient-dense leafy greens.

2 large eggs

¼ cup (60 ml) + 2 tablespoons (30 ml) ghee, butter, or duck fat, divided

14 ounces (400 g) smoked haddock or cod

½ medium (55 g/1.9 oz) yellow onion, diced

4 cups (480 g/16.9 oz) cauli-rice (page 14)

2 tablespoons (30 ml) lemon juice

1 tablespoon (6 g/0.2 oz) mild curry powder

½ cup (120 ml) coconut cream or heavy whipping cream

7 ounces (200 g) chard, collard greens, or spinach, roughly chopped

1 small (14 g/0.5 oz) mild chile pepper, sliced

2 tablespoons (8 g/0.3 oz) chopped parsley or cilantro

Salt and pepper, to taste

Cook the eggs until hard-boiled and set aside (see page 15 for instructions). Meanwhile, grease a large skillet or a casserole dish with 2 tablespoons (30 ml) of ghee. Add the smoked haddock and cook over high heat on both sides until opaque, about 2 minutes per side. Remove from the skillet. Once cool, break the fish into large flakes and set aside.

Grease the pan where you cooked the fish with the remaining ¼ cup (60 ml) of ghee. Add the onion and cook for 3 to 5 minutes, until fragrant. Add the cauli-rice, lemon juice, curry powder, and coconut cream. Cook for 7 to 8 minutes. Add the chard and cook for 1 minute, until wilted. Add the chile pepper, parsley, and flaked fish. Stir gently. Peel and quarter the eggs. Top with the quartered eggs, and season with salt and pepper. Eat immediately, or let it cool and store in the fridge.

NUTRITION FACTS PER SERVING:
Total carbs: 12.9 g / Fiber: 5.1 g / Net carbs: 7.8 g / Protein: 33.2 g / Fat: 35.7 g / Calories: 497 kcal
Macronutrient ratio: Calories from carbs (6%), protein (27%), fat (67%)

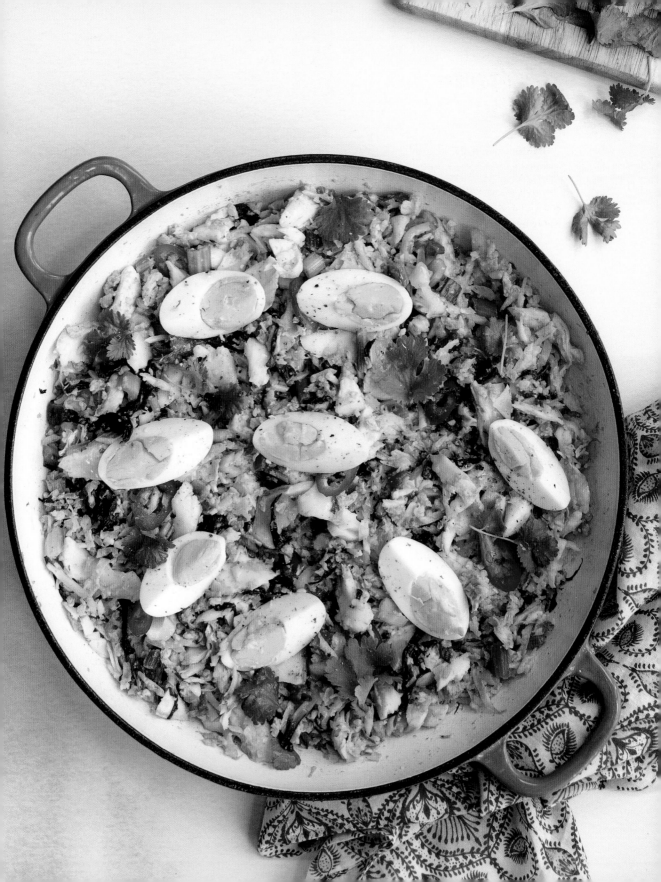

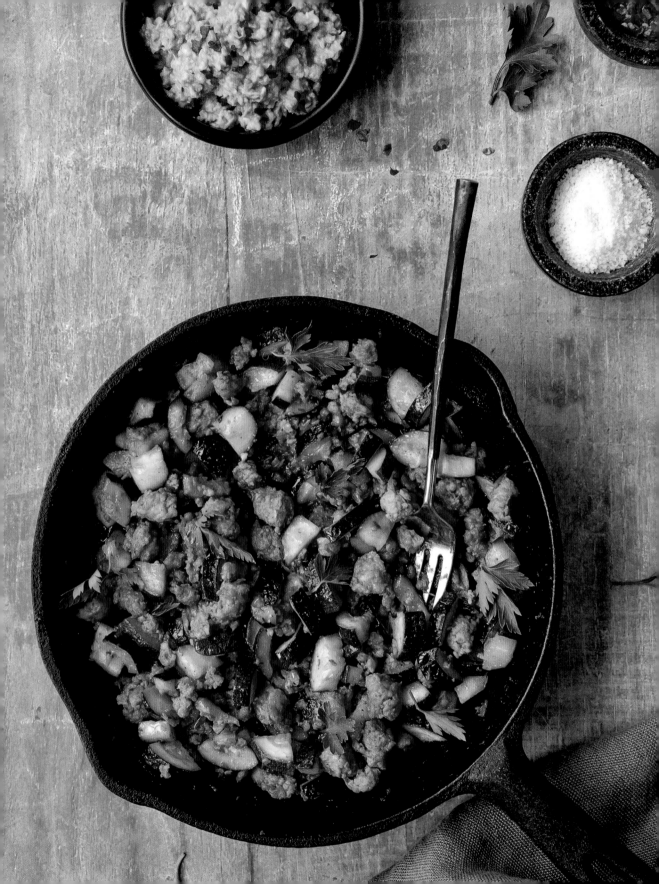

Harissa Pork & Zucchini Hash

SERVINGS: 2
HANDS-ON TIME: 10 minutes
OVERALL TIME: 15 minutes

Tired of eggs for breakfast? This easy skillet meal is packed with flavor and ideal for those days when you don't feel like eating eggs.

1 teaspoon ghee or duck fat

8 ounces (227 g) ground pork or gluten-free sausage meat

2 tablespoons (30 g/1.1 oz) harissa paste

1 medium (200 g/7.1 oz) zucchini, diced into ½-inch (1 cm) pieces

2 tablespoons (8 g/0.3 oz) fresh chopped parsley or cilantro

½ large (100 g/3.5 oz) avocado

2 teaspoons (10 ml) fresh lemon or lime juice

¼ small (20 g/0.7 oz) white onion, diced

½ clove garlic, minced

Salt, pepper, and red pepper flakes, to taste

Heat a medium skillet greased with ghee over medium-high heat. Add the pork and cook until browned. Add the harissa paste and zucchini. Reduce the heat to medium-low, cover with a lid, and cook for 5 to 7 minutes, until the zucchini is tender. Remove the lid and stir in the herbs. Set aside.

Place the avocado and lemon juice in a bowl, and mash with a fork. Stir in the onion and garlic. Season to taste with salt, pepper, and red pepper flakes. Serve with the harissa pork.

The zucchini hash can be stored in the fridge for up to 4 days. The mashed avocado is best eaten fresh but can be stored in a sealed jar in the fridge for 1 day.

TIP:
Swap the sausage meat for chorizo and skip the harissa paste. Use ground beef or ground chicken and swap the harissa for curry paste or Simple Pesto (page 16).

NUTRITION FACTS PER SERVING:
Total carbs: 12 g / Fiber: 5.8 g / Net carbs: 6.2 g / Protein: 22.1 g / Fat: 36 g / Calories: 452 kcal
Macronutrient ratio: Calories from carbs (6%), protein (20%), fat (74%)

Mexican Abundance Breakfast Bowl

SERVINGS: 2
HANDS-ON TIME: 15 minutes
OVERALL TIME: 20 minutes

This breakfast bowl is ultra-nutritious and satisfying. It's packed with flavor and looks so pretty too! If you make the chorizo cauli-rice in advance, you can make this tasty bowl in just 5 minutes. No more excuses!

3 ounces (85 g) Mexican chorizo or Spanish chorizo

2 cups (240 g/8.5 oz) cauli-rice (page 14)

¼ cup (60 g/2.1 oz) canned tomatoes or 4–6 cherry tomatoes, sliced

4 large eggs

Salt and pepper, to taste

1 tablespoon (15 ml) ghee, butter, or duck fat

1 medium (15 g/0.5 oz) spring onion, sliced

1 medium (150 g/5.3 oz) avocado, sliced

1 small (14 g/0.5 oz) jalapeño pepper, sliced

½ lime, cut into wedges

Fresh cilantro, to taste

1 tablespoon (15 ml) extra-virgin olive oil

Heat a large skillet over medium-high heat. Add the chorizo and cook for 2 minutes, until the juices are released and the sausage is browned. Add the cauli-rice and tomatoes and stir through. Cook for 5 to 7 minutes. Remove from the heat and divide between two serving bowls. Set the skillet aside.

TO MAKE THE SCRAMBLED EGGS: Crack the eggs in a mixing bowl. Season with salt and pepper and whisk with a fork. Grease the skillet with the ghee. Add the eggs and cook while stirring over medium-high heat for about 1 minute, until scrambled. Take off the heat and mix in the spring onion. Divide the scrambled eggs between the serving bowls.

To serve, add avocado, jalapeño pepper, lime wedges, and cilantro. Season with salt and pepper to taste, and drizzle with olive oil. Eat immediately. The chorizo cauli-rice and scrambled eggs can be stored in a sealed container in the fridge for up to 4 days.

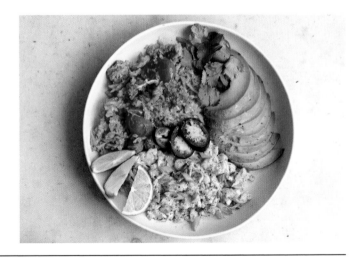

NUTRITION FACTS PER SERVING:
Total carbs: 16.9 g / Fiber: 8.9 g / Net carbs: 8 g / Protein: 23.6 g / Fat: 43.6 g / Calories: 540 kcal
Macronutrient ratio: Calories from carbs (6%), protein (18%), fat (76%)

Jalapeño Popper Breakfast Casserole

SERVINGS: 2
HANDS-ON TIME: 5 minutes
OVERALL TIME: 25 to 30 minutes

This easy breakfast casserole for two is packed with heat and flavor. It's easy to scale up and ideal for meal prep and freezing! If you don't like too much heat, use pickled jalapeño slices instead for a milder heat.

4 large eggs

¼ cup (60 ml) heavy whipping cream

3 tablespoons (45 g/1.5 oz) full-fat cream cheese

Pinch of black pepper

1 tablespoon (4 g/0.2 oz) fresh herbs such as cilantro or parsley

4 slices (57 g/2 oz) cooked bacon (see page 14), chopped

2 small (28 g/1 oz) jalapeño peppers, sliced

½ cup (57 g/2 oz) grated Cheddar cheese, divided

Optional: more jalapeño slices and hot sauce

Preheat the oven to 350°F (175°C) forced fan or 380°F (195°C) conventional.

In a bowl, whisk the eggs with the whipping cream, cream cheese, pepper, herbs, bacon, jalapeños, and half of the Cheddar. Pour the mixture into a small baking dish. Top the mixture with the reserved Cheddar cheese. Place the dish in the oven and bake for 20 to 25 minutes. Eat warm or cold, optionally topped with jalapeños and hot sauce. Store in the fridge for up to 4 days or freeze for up to 3 months.

TIP:
Can't find sugar-free hot sauce? If you want to make your own condiments, there are plenty of recipes on my blog at ketodietapp.com/blog.

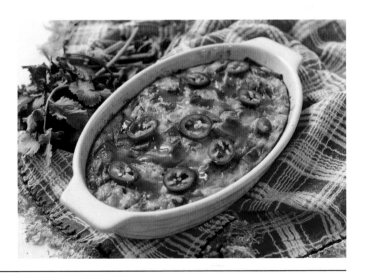

NUTRITION FACTS PER SERVING:
Total carbs: 4.2 g / Fiber: 0.6 g / Net carbs: 3.6 g / Protein: 29.8 g / Fat: 39.5 g / Calories: 486 kcal
Macronutrient ratio: Calories from carbs (3%), protein (25%), fat (72%)

Italian-Style Abundance Bowls

Making zucchini nests is easier than you think! What I love most about this recipe is the runny egg yolks. If you can find duck eggs, it's even better. They have bigger, deliciously creamy yolks!

1 tablespoon (15 ml) ghee or duck fat

2 pieces (130 g/4.6 oz) gluten-free Italian sausage

1 small (100 g/3.5 oz) zucchini, spiralized (see tip)

2 large chicken eggs or duck eggs

6 whole (60 g/2.1 oz) cherry tomatoes on the vine or 1 small tomato, halved

Salt, pepper, red pepper flakes, and fresh basil or herbs of choice, to taste

Optional: 1 tablespoon (15 g/0.5 oz) Simple Pesto (page 16), spooned on top of the zucchini nests

Heat a large skillet greased with ghee over medium heat. Place the sausages on one side and cook on all sides, until browned and cooked through.

Using the zucchini noodles, create two small nests by wrapping the noodles around your index and middle fingers to make a small well. Place the zucchini nests next to the sausages and crack in the eggs. Cook until the whites are opaque.

When the eggs are almost ready, place the tomatoes in the skillet and roast for a 2 to 3 minutes. Alternatively, you can serve them uncooked. Season to taste and serve immediately.

TIP:

To make zucchini noodles: Use a julienne peeler or a spiralizer to turn the zucchini into thin or wide "noodles." Chop the soft cores and add them to the noodles. Sprinkle the noodles with salt and let them sit for 10 minutes. Use a paper towel to pat them dry. Set aside.

NUTRITION FACTS PER SERVING:
Total carbs: 7.2 g / Fiber: 2.5 g / Net carbs: 4.7 g / Protein: 35.8 g / Fat: 48.2 g / Calories: 606 kcal
Macronutrient ratio: Calories from carbs (3%), protein (24%), fat (73%)

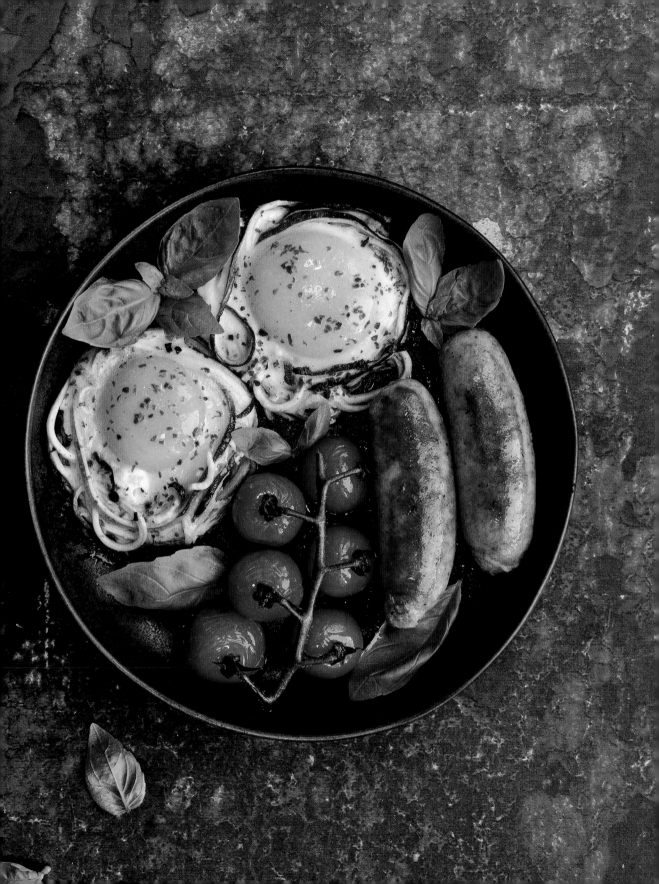

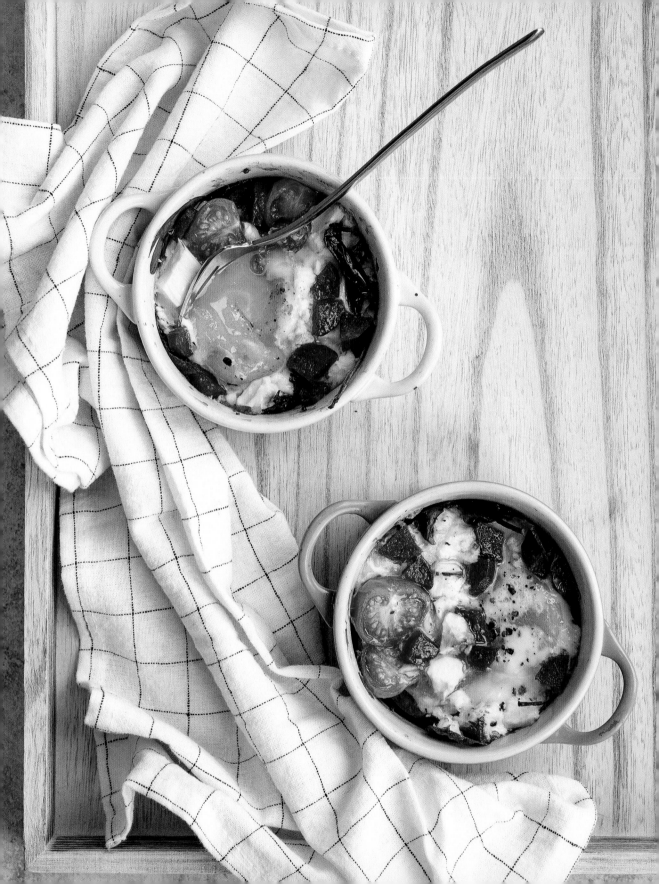

Single-Serve Baked Egg Pots

SERVINGS: 2
HANDS-ON TIME: 5 minutes
OVERALL TIME: 15 minutes

These breakfast egg pots are the perfect single-serve meal. I like mine with spinach, chorizo, and feta, but you can use any leafy greens, cheese, and any protein. Eat one serving as a light dish and two servings for a filling and nutritious breakfast.

1 cup (60 g/2.1 oz) fresh spinach

2 teaspoons (10 ml) extra-virgin olive oil

2 large eggs

2 ounces (57 g) diced Spanish chorizo

⅓ cup (50 g/1.8 oz) crumbled feta cheese

4 pieces (50 g/1.8 oz) cherry tomatoes, halved

Black pepper or red pepper flakes, to taste

Preheat the oven to 430°F (220°C) forced fan or 465°F (240°C) conventional.

Place the spinach in two 12-ounce (360 ml) ramekins or mugs. Drizzle each with a teaspoon of the olive oil. Crack an egg into each ramekin. Top with the chorizo, feta, and tomatoes. Place the ramekins in the oven and bake for 10 to 12 minutes, until the whites are set and the yolks are still runny. Season to taste and eat immediately.

TIPS:
• No time to cook? Use a microwave to cook for 1 to 2 minutes, until the whites are set.
• Swap the fresh spinach for frozen, thawed, and drained spinach. You can also use kale, collards, or chard.
• Swap the feta for soft goat's cheese or even grated Cheddar.
• Swap the Spanish chorizo for pepperoni, smoked salmon, sardines, or cooked diced chicken.

NUTRITION FACTS PER SERVING:
Total carbs: 3.4 g / Fiber: 0.9 g / Net carbs: 2.5 g / Protein: 17.3 g / Fat: 26.3 g / Calories: 323 kcal
Macronutrient ratio: Calories from carbs (3%), protein (22%), fat (75%)

Baked Cauliflower Pancakes

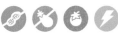

SERVINGS: 4 (8 pancakes total)
HANDS-ON TIME: 15 minutes
OVERALL TIME: 40 minutes

This is a new cool way to make savory pancakes! I like mine with crispy bacon slices and a touch of sugar-free maple syrup or simply with sliced avocado. You can even use these instead of bread in Eggs Benedict (page 26).

- 4 tablespoons (60 ml) ghee or duck fat, divided
- 1 small (450 g/1 lb.) cauliflower, riced (page14)
- 1¼ cups (140 g/5 oz) grated Cheddar cheese
- ¼ teaspoon salt, or to taste
- ¼ teaspoon pepper, or to taste
- 2 teaspoons (2 g/0.1 oz) onion powder
- 2 tablespoons (8 g/0.3 oz) chopped parsley
- 3 large eggs
- Optional: serve with crispy bacon slices or sliced avocado

Heat a large skillet greased with 2 tablespoons (30 ml) of ghee over medium-high heat. Add the cauli-rice and cook for 8 to 10 minutes, stirring frequently. Take off the heat and transfer to a mixing bowl. Add the Cheddar, salt, pepper, onion powder, parsley, and eggs. Mix to create a dough.

Preheat the oven 400°F (200°C) forced fan or 425°F (220°C) conventional. Line a baking sheet with parchment paper.

Use a ⅓-cup (80 ml) measuring cup to create 8 mounds and place them on the baking sheet (for 8 pancakes you will need 2 baking sheets). Using your hands, flatten each one until about ½ inch (1 cm) thick. Place in the oven and bake for 15 minutes. Remove from the oven, and brush with 1 tablespoon (15 ml) of ghee. Use a spatula to flip onto the other side and brush with the remaining 1 tablespoon (15 ml) of ghee. Place back in the oven and bake for 10 to 15 minutes.

Eat hot or cold and optionally serve with bacon or avocado. Store in a sealed jar in the fridge for up to 5 days.

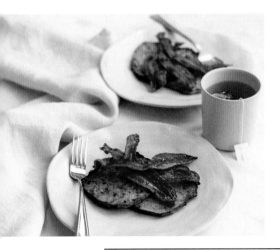

NUTRITION FACTS PER SERVING (2 PANCAKES):
Total carbs: 8.1 g / Fiber: 2.5 g / Net carbs: 5.6 g / Protein: 15.1 g / Fat: 30.7 g / Calories: 366 kcal
Macronutrient ratio: Calories from carbs (6%), protein (17%), fat (77%)

All-Day Breakfast Sausage Tray Bake

SERVINGS: 2
HANDS-ON TIME: 10 minutes
OVERALL TIME: 30 minutes

When it's too late for breakfast and too early for lunch, here comes the brunch! This simple tray bake is my breakfast staple on busy days. Beefsteak tomatoes work best for broiling because they contain fewer seeds, but even cherry tomatoes on the vine are a great option!

2 tablespoons (30 ml) ghee, duck fat, or olive oil, divided

10 ounces (285 g) gluten-free pork sausages

6 medium (85 g/3 oz) brown or white mushrooms

1 teaspoon dried Italian herbs, divided

3 cups (85 g/3 oz) roughly chopped chard, spinach, or kale

2 large eggs

1 large (200 g/7.1 oz) tomato, halved

Salt and pepper, to taste

Optional: fresh herbs of choice

Preheat the broiler to high, or preheat the oven to 430°F (220°C) forced fan or 465°F (240°C) conventional.

Grease a casserole dish or a deep baking tray with 1 teaspoon (5 ml) of ghee. Add the sausages and broil for 10 minutes, turning the sausages halfway through the time. Add the mushrooms top-side down, and sprinkle with ½ teaspoon of the dried herbs and 1 tablespoon (15 ml) of ghee. Bake for 5 minutes.

Add the chard and tomatoes and sprinkle with the remaining ½ teaspoon of herbs. Drizzle the tomatoes with the remaining ghee. The greens tend to burn, so it's best to move the chard below the sausages, mushrooms, and tomatoes. Crack the eggs on top of the greens and bake for 10 minutes, or until the whites are set and the yolks still runny. Seaon with salt and pepper. Optionally, sprinkle with fresh herbs of choice to taste. Eat immediately.

TIP:

Are you a one-meal-a-day (OMAD) eater? If you're the OMAD-style keto eater who practices intermittent fasting, this makes a great large meal! Simply serve as one meal or add more eggs or sausages to increase the protein and/or fat count.

PICTURED ON PAGE 19

NUTRITION FACTS PER SERVING:
Total carbs: 8.8 g / Fiber: 2.8 g / Net carbs: 6 g / Protein: 32.5 g / Fat: 45.6 g / Calories: 574 kcal
Macronutrient ratio: Calories from carbs (4%), protein (23%), fat (73%)

Breakfast Skillet Danish

SERVINGS: 2
HANDS-ON TIME: 10 minutes
OVERALL TIME: 30 minutes

Danish, soufflé, omelet, or pancake—there are many ways to describe this easy keto breakfast meal. It's a fluffy egg-based pastry with cheesecake filling and roasted strawberries. I call this heaven in a pan!

3 large eggs

⅔ cup (160 g/5.6 oz) full-fat cream cheese

1 teaspoon fresh lemon zest

½ teaspoon sugar-free vanilla extract

¼ cup (40 g/1.4 oz) powdered erythritol or Swerve, divided (plus more for serving; optional)

½ teaspoon lemon juice

⅓ cup (33 g/1.2 oz) almond flour, or 1½ tablespoon (12 g/0.4 oz) more coconut flour

2 tablespoons (16 g/0.6 oz) coconut flour

1 tablespoon (15 ml) ghee or virgin coconut oil

2 medium (57 g/2 oz) fresh strawberries, sliced

Preheat the oven to 300°F (150°C) forced fan or 340°F (170°C) conventional.

To make the filling: Separate the egg whites from the egg yolks. Combine the cream cheese with 1 egg yolk, the lemon zest, vanilla, and 2 tablespoons (20 g/0.7 oz) of the erythritol.

Add the lemon juice to the bowl with the egg whites. Using an electric mixer or a hand whisk, start whisking the egg whites and add in the remaining 2 tablespoons (20 g/0.7 oz) of erythritol. Keep beating until stiff peaks form. Fold the remaining 2 egg yolks into the mixture using a silicone spatula. Sift in the almond flour and coconut flour and gently combine with the egg white mixture without deflating it.

Grease an ovenproof 8-inch (20 cm) skillet with ghee and heat it over medium heat. Pour in the fluffy pancake mixture, and then cook on low heat for 1 minute. Spoon the filling in the middle of the pancake and spread evenly, leaving about an inch (2.5 cm) on the sides.

Add the sliced strawberries, transfer the skillet to the oven, and bake for 20 to 25 minutes, until the pancake is golden and the filling is set. Optionally, dust with powdered sweetener. Eat warm or cold.

This recipe makes two regular breakfast servings or up to four dessert servings. Store in the fridge for up to 3 days.

TIP:

Need to cut the carb count? Swap the strawberries for blackberries or simply skip the fruit topping.

NUTRITION FACTS PER SERVING (½ PANCAKE):
Total carbs: 12.3 g / Fiber: 3.9 g / Net carbs: 8.4 g / Protein: 20.2 g / Fat: 47.1 g / Calories: 516 kcal
Macronutrient ratio: Calories from carbs (6%), protein (15%), fat (79%

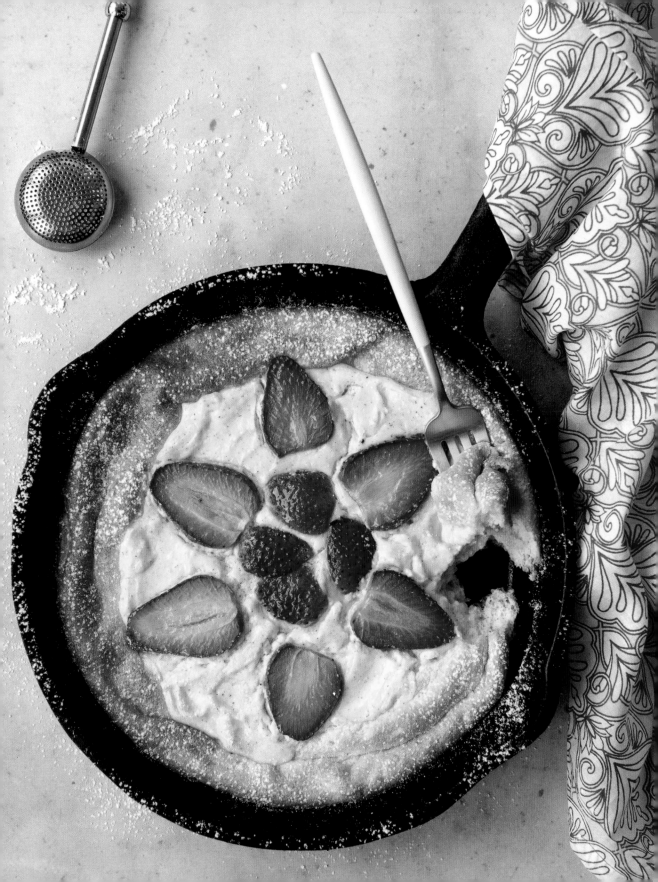

Cookie Dough Overnight Noatmeal

SERVINGS: 4
HANDS-ON TIME: 5 minutes
OVERALL TIME: 30 minutes

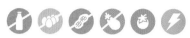

These cookie dough–flavored jars are a tasty alternative to breakfast oatmeal. All the flavors of your favorite overnight oatmeal with none of the carbs.

½ cup (120 ml) coconut cream or heavy whipping cream

1 cup (240 ml) unsweetened almond or cashew milk

1 tablespoon (16 g/0.6 oz) almond butter

¼ cup (40 g/1.4 oz) powdered erythritol or Swerve

½ teaspoon ground cinnamon

1 teaspoon fresh lemon zest

Pinch of salt

¼ cup (32 g/1.1 oz) chia seeds

½ cup (57 g/2 oz) chopped pecans or walnuts

¼ cup (50 g/1.8 oz) 90% dark chocolate chips or chopped chocolate (Use at least 85% chocolate or sugar-free chocolate.)

Place the coconut cream, almond milk, almond butter, erythritol, cinnamon, lemon zest, and salt in a blender. Pulse until smooth and then pour into a bowl. Add the chia seeds, and set aside for 20 to 30 minutes, or overnight.

To assemble the dish: Divide the prepared chia mixture among four jars. Just before serving, top with the pecans and chocolate chips. The chia pudding can be stored in the fridge for up to 4 days, separately from the toppings. (The toppings would get soggy if kept together with the pudding.)

TIPS:

• Love smoothies? This recipe makes a delicious cookie dough–flavored smoothie! Simply skip the chia seeds and pecans and add collagen to the blender (1 to 2 tablespoons per smoothie).

• Are you nut-free? Swap the almond milk for any seed milk or simply use water. Instead of almond butter, use coconut butter or sunflower seed butter. Finally, swap the pecans for toasted coconut flakes.

• Low-carb sweeteners can be used to taste. You can skip the sweetener altogether or use other options, such as monk fruit or stevia drops.

PICTURED ON PAGE 19

NUTRITION FACTS PER SERVING:
Total carbs: 11.7 g / Fiber: 6.5 g / Net carbs: 5.2 g / Protein: 6.4 g / Fat: 33.2 g / Calories: 345 kcal
Macronutrient ratio: Calories from carbs (6%), protein (7%), fat (87%)

Chocolate Pancakes

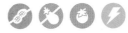

SERVINGS: 4 (8 small pancakes total)
HANDS-ON TIME: 15 minutes
OVERALL TIME: 15 minutes

Following a low-carb diet doesn't mean you have to say no to all treats. So why not have a dessert for breakfast? These chocolate pancakes are a great way to start the day if you crave something sweet. Serve with fluffy whipped cream and berries.

4 large eggs

⅓ cup (85 g/3 oz) full-fat cream cheese or ricotta, at room temperature

1 teaspoon sugar-free vanilla extract or ½ teaspoon ground cinnamon

¼ cup (50 g/1.8 oz) granulated erythritol or Swerve

¼ cup (22 g/0.8 oz) cacao powder or Dutch-process cocoa powder

1 cup (100 g/3.5 oz) almond flour or ground sunflower seeds

1 teaspoon gluten-free baking powder

2 tablespoons (30 ml) ghee or coconut oil, or as needed for frying

Crack the eggs into a bowl. Add the cream cheese and vanilla and whisk until well combined. In another bowl, combine the erythritol, cacao powder, almond flour, and baking powder. Add the dry ingredients to the bowl with the eggs and mix well again.

Grease a large pan with ghee and heat over medium-low heat. Using a ¼-cup (60 ml) measuring cup or ladle, gradually cook 8 small pancakes. (You can use pancake molds to create perfect shapes.) Cook each pancake for about 3 minutes, or until the tops start to firm up. Flip the pancakes over and cook for 1 minute.

Store leftover pancakes in a sealed container in the fridge for up to 5 days or freeze for up to 3 months.

TIPS:
- Serve with butter, full-fat yogurt, whipped cream (optionally whipped with some cacao powder and sweetener), or low-carb syrup such as yacon or monk fruit syrup.
- Instead of baking powder, you can use a combination of baking soda and cream of tartar. To do that, use the following conversion: 1 teaspoon baking powder = ¼ teaspoon of baking soda + ½ teaspoon of cream of tartar (or ½ teaspoon of lemon juice).
- Are you nut-free? Simply skip the almond flour and add ⅓ cup (40 g/1.4 oz) coconut flour plus ¼ cup (60 g/2.1 oz) cream cheese.

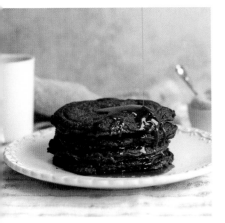

NUTRITION FACTS PER SERVING (2 PANCAKES):
Total carbs: 9.8 g / Fiber: 4.5 g / Net carbs: 5.3 g / Protein: 14.2 g / Fat: 32.1 g / Calories: 358 kcal
Macronutrient ratio: Calories from carbs (6%), protein (15%), fat (79%)

Coconut Chia Granola Crunch

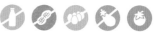

SERVINGS: 10
HANDS-ON TIME: 10 minutes
OVERALL TIME: 1 hour + cooling

This grain-free cinnamon granola crunch is a tasty breakfast and a convenient travel-friendly snack. You can easily scale it up and keep it in a sealed container for weeks!

1¼ cups (94 g/3.3 oz) unsweetened shredded coconut

½ cup (76 g/2.7 oz) chia seeds

2½ cups (150 g/5.3 oz) flaked coconut

1 tablespoon (15 ml) virgin coconut oil

½ cup (120 ml) water

¼ cup (50 g/1.8 oz) granulated erythritol or Swerve

½ cup (125 g/4.4 oz) coconut butter or almond butter

1 teaspoon sugar-free vanilla extract

2 teaspoons (5 g/0.2 oz) ground cinnamon

¼ teaspoon salt

½ cup (90 g/3.2 oz) 90% dark chocolate chips (Use at least 85% chocolate or sugar-free chocolate.)

Combine all the ingredients, apart from the chocolate chips, in a mixing bowl. Set it aside for about 15 minutes.

Meanwhile, preheat the oven to 285°F (140°C) forced fan or 320°F (160°C) conventional.

Spread the mixture on a baking tray and transfer to the oven. Bake for 45 to 60 minutes, mixing the granola once or twice. Remove from the oven and let the granola cool down. It may feel soft when you first remove it from the oven but will crisp up as it cools.

Once it's completely cool, add the chocolate chips. Transfer to a jar or a sealed container. Store at room temperature for up to 1 month. Serve with coconut milk, almond milk, or full-fat yogurt.

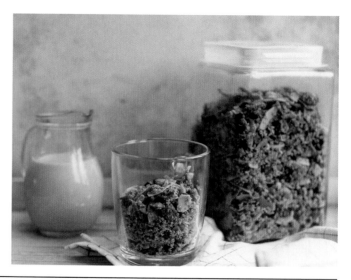

NUTRITION FACTS PER SERVING (½ CUP/57 G/2 OZ):
Total carbs: 13.8 g / Fiber: 9.3 g / Net carbs: 4.5 g / Protein: 6.1 g / Fat: 28.2 g / Calories: 319 kcal
Macronutrient ratio: Calories from carbs (6%), protein (8%), fat (86%)

Creamy Breakfast Hot Chocolate

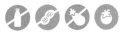

SERVINGS: 1
HANDS-ON TIME: 5 minutes
OVERALL TIME: 5 minutes

If you like bulletproof coffee, you will love this one. And don't worry, the egg yolks won't scramble. Instead, they will make this breakfast drink creamy and nutritious!

1 cup (240 ml) boiling water

2 tablespoons (11 g/0.4 oz) cacao powder or Dutch-process cocoa powder

¼ teaspoon sugar-free vanilla extract or ground cinnamon

2 tablespoons (28 g/1 oz) unsalted butter or virgin coconut oil

5 drops liquid stevia, or any low-carb sweetener, to taste

3 egg yolks

Place all the ingredients in a blender and process until smooth, creamy, and frothy on top. Pour into a serving glass and drink immediately.

TIPS:

• Swap hot water for unsweetened almond milk or cashew milk.

• Swap hot water for hot coffee or simply add a teaspoon of instant coffee powder for a mocha-flavored breakfast drink.

• Add 1 to 2 tablespoons (15 to 30 ml) of heavy whipping cream or coconut cream.

• For extra protein, add 1 to 2 tablespoons (7 to 14 g/0.3 to 0.6 oz) of collagen powder.

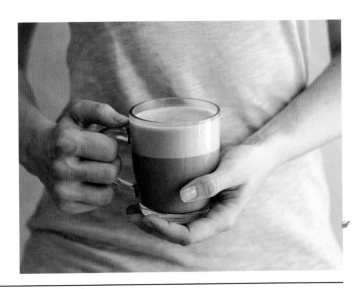

NUTRITION FACTS PER SERVING:
Total carbs: 8.1 g / Fiber: 4 g / Net carbs: 4.1 g / Protein: 10.4 g / Fat: 38.1 g / Calories: 395 kcal
Macronutrient ratio: Calories from carbs (4%), protein (10%), fat (86%)

No-tella Breakfast Smoothie

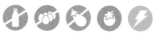

SERVINGS: 1
HANDS-ON TIME: 5 minutes
OVERALL TIME: 5 minutes

Hazelnut butter is the key ingredient that gives this deliciously creamy, nutritious smoothie a Nutella-like flavor. If you can't get hold of roasted hazelnut butter, simply use roasted hazelnuts—just make sure they are peeled, as the skins tend to leave a bitter aftertaste.

2 large eggs

3 tablespoons (45 ml) heavy whipping cream

½ cup (120 ml) unsweetened almond milk or hazelnut milk

¼ cup (28 g/1 oz) roasted peeled hazelnuts, or 2 tablespoons (28 g/1 oz) roasted hazelnut butter

1 tablespoon (5 g/0.2 oz) cacao powder or Dutch-process cocoa powder

3–5 drops liquid stevia or any low-carb sweetener, to taste

¼ teaspoon sugar-free vanilla extract

Optional: ice cubes for the smoothie, whipped cream, and cacao powder for topping

Place all the ingredients in a blender (optionally with ice cubes). Process until smooth, creamy, and frothy on top. Pour into a serving glass and drink immediately.

TIPS:

• Are you dairy-free? Swap the whipping cream for coconut cream.

• Are you egg-free? Instead of eggs, you can use 2 to 4 tablespoons (14 to 28 g/0.6 to 1.2 oz) of collagen powder or whey protein powder.

• Worried about using raw eggs? See the note on page 16 for information on pasteurizing eggs.

NUTRITION FACTS PER SERVING:
Total carbs: 10.7 g / Fiber: 5.1 g / Net carbs: 5.6 g / Protein: 19.3 g / Fat: 46 g / Calories: 518 kcal
Macronutrient ratio: Calories from carbs (4%), protein (15%), fat (81%)

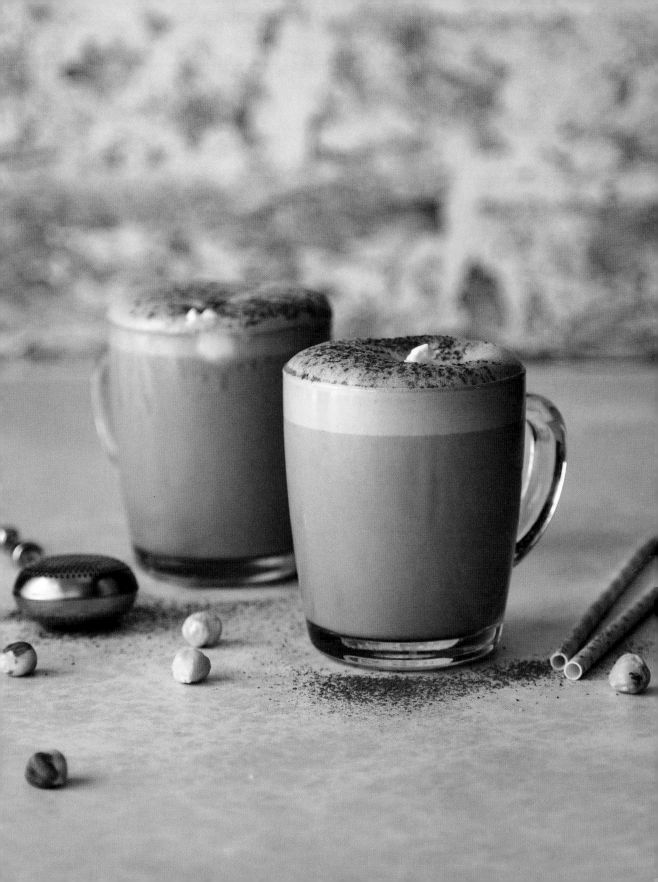

Chapter 3

Snacks

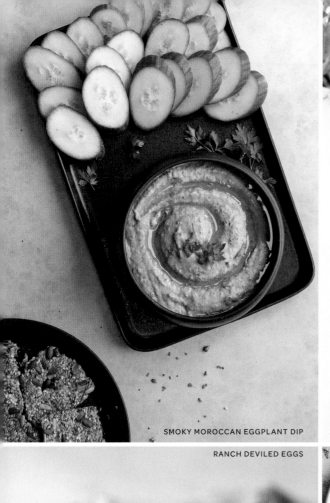

SMOKY MOROCCAN EGGPLANT DIP

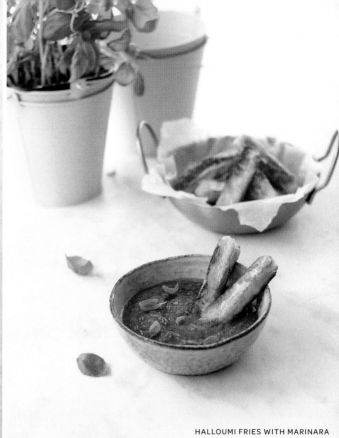

HALLOUMI FRIES WITH MARINARA

RANCH DEVILED EGGS

CHEESY SPINACH & ARTICHOKE DIP

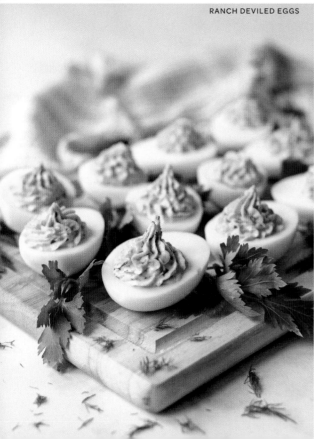

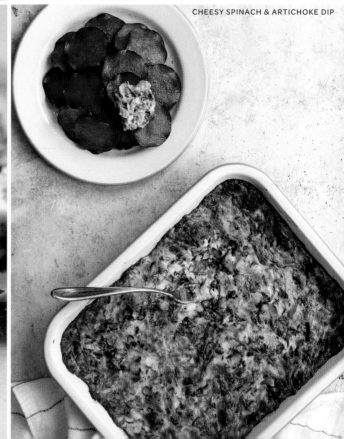

Cheesy Pepperoni Twists

SERVINGS: 8
HANDS-ON TIME: 10 minutes
OVERALL TIME: 20 minutes

Five ingredients. That's all you need to make these crispy pepperoni twists! Nibble them on their own, smother them in mashed avocado, or dunk them in a bowl of homemade marinara (page 55).

1½ cups (170 g/6 oz) shredded
   low-moisture mozzarella
⅔ cup (66 g/2.3 oz) almond flour
3 ounces (85 g) chopped pepperoni or
   Spanish chorizo
4 tablespoons (20 g/0.8 oz) grated
   Parmesan cheese, divided
Red pepper flakes, to taste

Preheat the oven to 400°F (200°C) forced fan or 425°F (220°C) conventional. Line a baking sheet with parchment paper.

Melt the mozzarella in the microwave for 60 to 90 seconds (or melt on the stove over low heat while stirring), checking halfway through. Mix and add in the almond flour. Stir until well combined.

Roll out the dough thinly between two sheets of parchment paper or use a nonstick mat and nonstick rolling pin. When rolled out, the dough should be about 16 x 12 inches (40 x 30 cm).

Sprinkle with pepperoni and half of the Parmesan. Fold the side of the dough without the pepperoni on it over to the other side, covering the filing. Use a sharp knife or a pizza cutter to cut the dough into 8 strips, each one about 1½ inches (4 cm) thick. Twist the strips a few times and press down on the ends to keep them closed.

Place the twists on the parchment-lined baking sheet, then sprinkle with red pepper flakes and the remaining Parmesan. Bake for 10 to 12 minutes, until golden brown. Eat warm or cold, and store in a sealed contained in the fridge for up to 5 days.

TIP:

Are you nut-free? You can easily convert this recipe by adding 2 ounces (57 g) of full-fat cream cheese in the shredded mozzarella before microwaving it, and then swapping the almond flour for either 6 tablespoons (48 g/1.7 oz) of coconut flour or 8 tablespoons (57 g/2 oz) of flax meal.

NUTRITION FACTS PER SERVING (1 TWIST):
Total carbs: 2.9 g / Fiber: 0.9 g / Net carbs: 2 g / Protein: 10.1 g / Fat: 13.9 g / Calories: 174 kcal
Macronutrient ratio: Calories from carbs (5%), protein (23%), fat (72%)

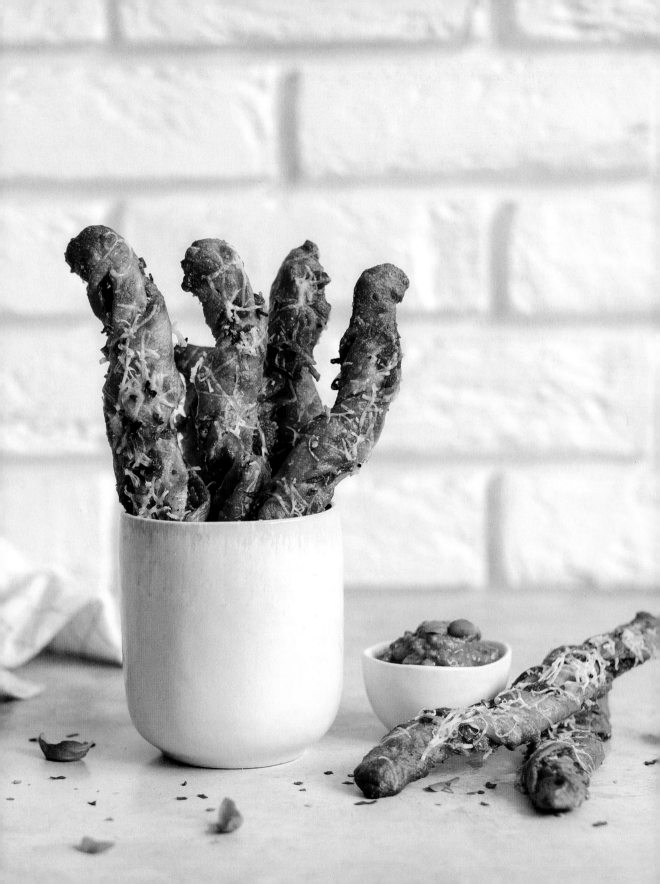

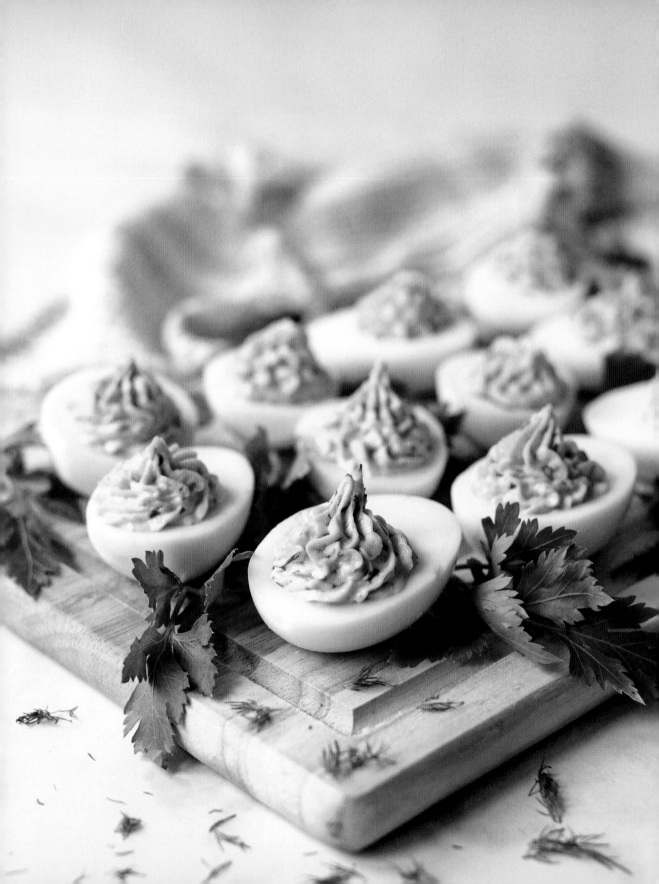

Ranch Deviled Eggs

SERVINGS: 6
HANDS-ON TIME: 10 minutes
OVERALL TIME: 20 minutes

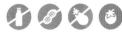

I always keep some hard-boiled eggs in the fridge. They are essential for meal prep, and they make life easier for any busy cook! Then it takes just a few minutes to assemble a tasty, nutritious snack.

6 large eggs

3 tablespoons (45 g/1.5 oz) mayonnaise (page 16)

2 tablespoons (30 g/1.1 oz) sour cream, or more mayonnaise

1 tablespoon (8 g/0.3 oz) ranch seasoning

Black pepper and fresh herbs (parsley, dill, or chives), to taste

Hard-boil the eggs (see page 15). Cut the eggs in half and carefully—without breaking the egg whites—spoon the egg yolks into a bowl. Set the whites aside. Mix the egg yolks with the mayo, sour cream, and ranch seasoning. Use a spoon or a piping bag to fill the egg white halves with the mixture. Season with black pepper and sprinkle with fresh herbs. Store in a sealed container in the fridge for up to 2 days.

TIPS:

• To make your own ranch seasoning, simply use: ½ teaspoon each of garlic powder, onion powder, dried parsley, dried dill, dried chives, and salt. This will yield just 1 tablespoon needed in this recipe.

• Deviled eggs are incredibly versatile! Simply swap the ranch seasoning with everything bagel seasoning (page 21), Simple Pesto (page 16), harissa paste, smoky chipotle chile paste, or Thai curry paste.

NUTRITION FACTS PER SERVING (2 DEVILED EGGS):
Total carbs: 1.1 g / Fiber: 0.1 g / Net carbs: 1 g / Protein: 6.6 g / Fat: 12 g / Calories: 139 kcal
Macronutrient ratio: Calories from carbs (3%), protein (19%), fat (78%)

Cheese Crisps Two Ways

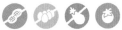

SERVINGS: 4
HANDS-ON TIME: 5 minutes
OVERALL TIME: 15 minutes

These three-ingredient cheese crisps are a fun snack or appetizer. They are travel-friendly and great for lunch boxes. Serve them with any high-fat dip, such as guacamole, Smoky Moroccan Eggplant Dip (page 56) or Simple Pesto (page 16).

PARMESAN CHEESE CRISPS

1 cup (90 g/3.2 oz) grated Parmesan cheese

1 tablespoon (4 g/0.2 oz) chopped thyme or 1 teaspoon dried thyme

4 pieces (14 g/0.5 oz) sun-dried tomatoes or olives

CHEDDAR CHEESE CRISPS

1 cup (113 g/4 oz) grated Cheddar cheese

1 small (14 g/0.5 oz) fresh jalapeño pepper, sliced or pickled jalapeños

1 ounce (28 g) Spanish chorizo or pepperoni, sliced

Preheat the oven to 410°F (210°C) forced fan or 450°F (230°C) conventional. Line a baking sheet with parchment paper.

Divide the cheese into 8 individual mounds and place them on the baking sheet. Make sure to leave enough space (ideally 2 inches/5 cm) between them, as the cheese will spread. Top each mound with the toppings.

Transfer to the oven and cook for 7 to 10 minutes, until the cheese is melted and starting to crisp around the edges.

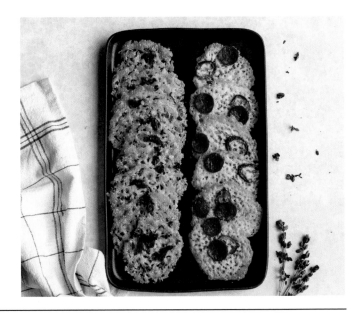

NUTRITION FACTS PER SERVING (2 PARMESAN/CHEDDAR CHEESE CRISPS):
Total carbs: 1.6/1.3 g / Fiber: 0.2/0.2 g / Net carbs: 1.4/1.1 g / Protein: 8.2/8.2 g / Fat: 6.3/12.2 g /
Calories: 97/148 kcal
Macronutrient ratio: Calories from carbs (6/3%), protein (35/22%), fat (59/75%)

Halloumi Fries with Marinara

SERVINGS: 4
HANDS-ON TIME: 15 minutes
OVERALL TIME: 15 minutes

 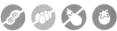

This is such a simple yet delicious keto snack. I can't imagine a summer barbecue without grilled or fried Halloumi fries! Just remember to eat them hot, as cold Halloumi gets rubbery.

1 pack (250 g/8.8 oz) Halloumi cheese
1 tablespoon (15 ml) ghee or olive oil
½ cup (120 ml) sugar-free marinara
sauce (see tip below)

Cut the Halloumi into 8 "fries," each about ¾ inch (2 cm) thick. Heat a large skillet greased with ghee over medium-high heat. Cook the Halloumi fries in batches, turning them to cook on all sides. At first, they will be hard to turn but once they develop a crispy golden crust, it's time to turn them.

Serve hot with marinara sauce. Halloumi fries are best eaten immediately but can be stored in the fridge for up to 3 days and reheated before serving.

TIPS:

• To make your own sugar-free Marinara: Place 1 cup (150 g/5.3 oz) chopped tomatoes, ½ cup (20 g/0.7 oz) fresh basil, 2 cloves garlic, 1 small (30 g/1.1 oz) shallot or white onion, ¼ cup (60 g/2.1 oz) tomato paste, ¼ cup (60 ml) extra-virgin olive oil, ¼ teaspoon salt, and black pepper to taste in a blender. Pulse until smooth.

• For a delicious change from marinara, try these with guacamole or Simple Pesto (page 16).

PICTURED ON PAGE 49

NUTRITION FACTS PER SERVING (2 FRIES + 2 TABLESPOONS [30 ML] MARINARA SAUCE):
Total carbs: 3 g / Fiber: 0.4 g / Net carbs: 2.6 g / Protein: 12.8 g / Fat: 25.5 g / Calories: 290 kcal
Macronutrient ratio: Calories from carbs (4%), protein (18%), fat (78%)

Smoky Moroccan Eggplant Dip

SERVINGS: 8 (about 2 cups [450 g])
HANDS-ON TIME: 10 minutes
OVERALL TIME: 1 hour

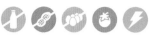

This is my favorite twist on baba ghanoush, an eggplant-based Middle Eastern dip. It's packed with flavor and extra heat from harissa!

2 large (750 g/1.7) eggplants (This will yield about 1.3 pounds [600 g] edible parts.)

¼ cup (60 ml) extra-virgin olive oil, divided

¼ cup (63 g/2.2 oz) tahini

2 cloves garlic, crushed

1 tablespoon (15 g/0.5 oz) harissa paste

½ teaspoon cumin powder

3 tablespoons (45 ml) lemon juice

2 tablespoons (8 g/0.3 oz) chopped parsley

Salt and pepper, to taste

Preheat the oven to 430°F (220°C) forced fan or 465°F (240°C) conventional.

Place the whole eggplants on a baking tray and bake for 40 to 50 minutes. They will get wrinkly and very soft inside when they are done. Remove from the oven and leave them to cool down enough to handle. Slit the eggplants and scoop the flesh out into a food processor, leaving the excess juice in the tray. Discard the skins, stems, and excess juices.

Place the remaining ingredients in a food processor—reserving 1 tablespoon (15 ml) of olive oil for topping. Pulse until smooth. Store covered in the fridge for up to 5 days. Drizzle with the remaining 1 tablespoon (15 ml) oil before serving.

TIPS:

• If you prefer your dip chunky, instead of using a food processor, mix all the ingredients apart from the eggplants in a bowl, then add the eggplant flesh and mash using a fork.

• Serve with crispy veggies, such as peppers, carrots, and cucumber, or with flaxseed crackers. You can find loads of recipes, including my Keto Naan Flat Bread and Multiseed Keto Crackers, on my blog at ketodietapp.com/blog!

PICTURED ON PAGE 49

NUTRITION FACTS PER SERVING (¼ CUP/57 G/2 OZ):
Total carbs: 7.1 g / Fiber: 3.2 g / Net carbs: 3.9 g / Protein: 2.3 g / Fat: 11.4 g / Calories: 132 kcal
Macronutrient ratio: Calories from carbs (12%), protein (7%), fat (81%)

Cheesy Spinach & Artichoke Dip

SERVINGS: 16 (about 4 cups [900 g])
HANDS-ON TIME: 5 minutes
OVERALL TIME: 30 minutes

An all-time favorite dip that can easily be eaten as a cheesy snack or as part of a light meal, this is my take on the popular recipe. I skipped the mayo and added extra cheese for a super-creamy result. It's also easy to scale up or down—so you can make just as much as you need!

8 ounces (227 g) frozen spinach, thawed and squeezed dry (weight excludes water squeezed out)

8 ounces (227 g) canned artichoke hearts, chopped

8 ounces (227 g) full-fat cream cheese

½ cup (115 g/4.1 oz) sour cream or full-fat yogurt

1½ cups (170 g/6 oz) grated mozzarella cheese

1 cup (113 g/4 oz) grated Cheddar or Swiss cheese

½ cup (45 g/1.5 oz) grated Parmesan cheese

2 cloves garlic, minced

Optional: dried Italian herbs and pepper, to taste

Preheat the oven to 355°F (180°C) forced fan or 400°F (200°C) conventional.

Place all the ingredients in a bowl and mix until combined. Transfer the mixture to a baking dish and spread and flatten with a spatula. Bake for 20 to 30 minutes, until golden, bubbly, and crisp, turning the dish after 10 to 15 minutes.

Serve warm, or let it cool down and refrigerate for up to 5 days. Microwave or reheat in the oven before serving.

TIP:

Serve with crispy bacon or with pepperoni slices baked at 355°F (180°C) forced fan or 400°F (200°C) conventional for about 10 minutes, turning the slices halfway through the cooking time. You can also eat this dip with flaxseed crackers (aka "flackers") or make your own. You can find loads of recipes, such as my Keto Garlic Bread and Tortilla Chips, at ketodietapp.com/blog.

PICTURED ON PAGE 49

NUTRITION FACTS PER SERVING (¼ CUP/57 G/2 OZ DIP):
Total carbs: 4 g / Fiber: 1.2 g / Net carbs: 2.8 g / Protein: 7.3 g / Fat: 10.7 g / Calories: 132 kcal
Macronutrient ratio: Calories from carbs (8%), protein (21%), fat (71%)

Chapter 4

Sides

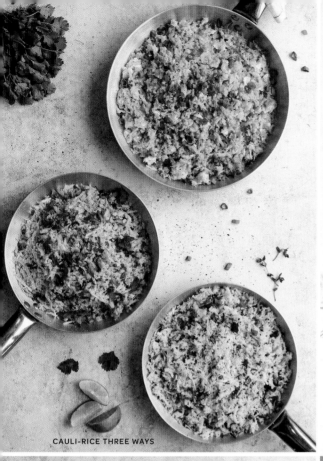

CAULI-RICE THREE WAYS

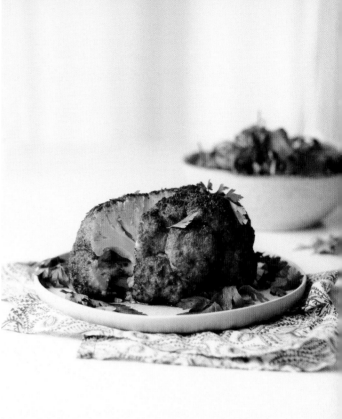

WHOLE ROASTED CAULIFLOWER TWO WAYS

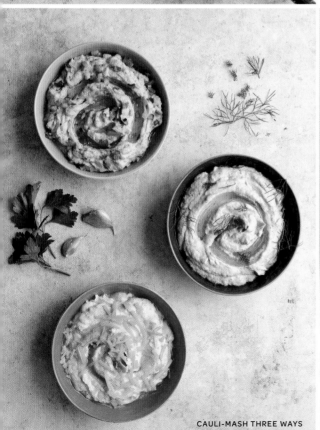

CAULI-MASH THREE WAYS

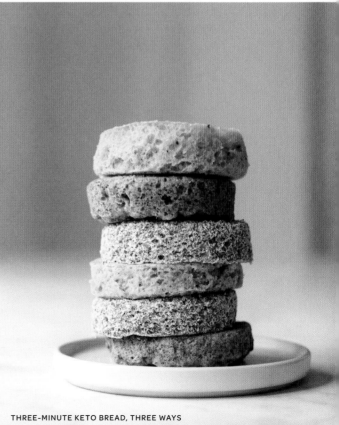

THREE-MINUTE KETO BREAD, THREE WAYS

Whole Roasted Cauliflower Two Ways

SERVINGS: 6
HANDS-ON TIME: 5 minutes
OVERALL TIME: 1 hour

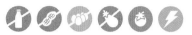

I love the idea of marinating and baking whole cauliflower because it's so simple yet impressive if you want to make this for a family gathering. I serve mine as a side or even as a light veggie meal with Homemade Marinara (page 55), Salsa Verde (page 103), Cucumber Raita (page 138), or Simple Pesto (page 16).

1 large (1 kg/2.2 lb.) cauliflower
½ teaspoon salt, or to taste
¼ teaspoon black pepper, or to taste

SPICY INDIAN
¼ cup (60 ml) ghee, olive oil, or duck fat
1 tablespoon (6 g/0.2 oz) garam masala
1 teaspoon paprika
1 teaspoon turmeric powder
1 teaspoon ground cumin

HERBY ITALIAN
2 tablespoons (30 ml) extra-virgin olive oil
¼ cup (60 g/2.1 oz) pesto (page 16)
1 tablespoon (15 ml) fresh lemon juice

Preheat the oven to 400°F (200°C) forced fan or 425°F (220°C) conventional.

Remove the tough outer leaves of the cauliflower. Mix the seasoning of choice and add salt and pepper. Rub the mixture all over the cauliflower and place in a snug-fitting baking dish or an ovenproof skillet. Add about ⅓ cup (80 ml) of water to the skillet.

Bake for 40 to 45 minutes, basting the cauliflower once or twice. Remove from the oven and let it cool down for 10 minutes. Slice and serve warm. Store in the fridge for up to 3 days.

TIPS:
• To boost the flavor, let the cauliflower marinate for an hour, or cover and place in the fridge to marinate overnight.
• Try this with harissa paste, Thai curry paste, or ranch seasoning by mixing ½ cup (115 g/4.1 oz) of sour cream or full-fat yogurt with our ranch seasoning on page 53.

NUTRITION FACTS PER SERVING (1/6TH SPICY INDIAN/HERBY ITALIAN):
Total carbs: 9.4/9.1 g / Fiber: 3.8/3.6 g / Net carbs: 5.6/5.5 g / Protein: 3.4/3.5 g / Fat: 10.7/11.6 g / Calories: 138/143 kcal
Macronutrient ratio: Calories from carbs (17/16%), protein (10/10%), fat (73/74%)

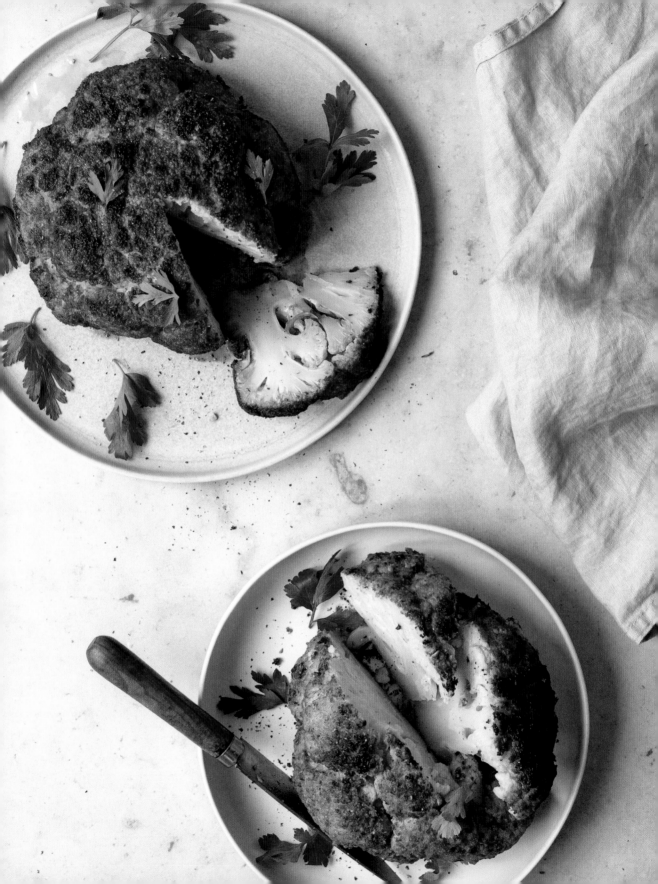

Browned Butter Asparagus

SERVINGS: 4
HANDS-ON TIME: 5 minutes
OVERALL TIME: 15 minutes

If you've never tried brown butter veggies, you are in for a treat! The caramelized flavor of the butter pairs perfectly with acidic vinegar and fragrant garlic. A simple-yet-delicious keto side in under fifteen minutes!

1.3 pounds (600 g) trimmed
asparagus spears

¼ teaspoon salt, or to taste

¼ teaspoon pepper, or to taste

1 tablespoon (15 ml) ghee or olive oil

3 tablespoons (45 g/1.5 oz) unsalted
butter

1 tablespoon (15 ml) coconut aminos
or tamari

1 teaspoon balsamic vinegar

1 clove garlic, minced

Preheat the oven to 400°F (200°C) forced fan or 425°F (220°C) conventional.

Place the asparagus in a large baking dish. Season with salt and pepper, and drizzle with ghee. Bake for 8 to 15 minutes. Thick asparagus spears may take up to 15 minutes; you can always cut them in half to make thinner spears. Remove from the oven and set aside.

Meanwhile, make the brown butter. Place the butter in a small saucepan and cook over medium heat for 3 to 5 minutes, until the milk solids start to brown. Then take off the heat and add the remaining ingredients. Pour evenly over the asparagus. Serve warm or refrigerate for up to 3 days. Reheat before serving.

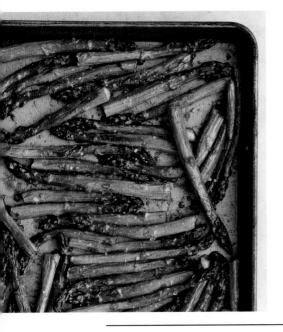

NUTRITION FACTS PER SERVING:
Total carbs: 6.6 g / Fiber: 3.2 g / Net carbs: 3.4 g / Protein: 3.5 g / Fat: 12.6 g / Calories: 144 kcal
Macronutrient ratio: Calories from carbs (10%), protein (10%), fat (80%)

Cauli-Rice Three Ways

SERVINGS: 5 (Egg Fried Cauli-Rice),
4 (Italian and Southwest Cauli-Rice)
HANDS-ON TIME: 15 minutes   **OVERALL TIME**: 15 to 20 minutes

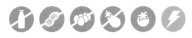

Cauliflower rice is a low-carb staple, but let's face it—plain grated cauliflower can get repetitive. So why not pack it with flavor from herbs and spices? Here are three examples of a tasty low-carb side dish that is anything but boring!

1 medium (720 g/1.6 lb.) cauliflower

EGG FRIED CAULI-RICE

3 tablespoons (45 ml) ghee or olive oil, divided

3 large eggs

Salt and pepper, to taste

2 medium (30 g/1.1 oz) spring onions, chopped

1 clove garlic, minced

2 tablespoons (30 ml) coconut aminos or tamari sauce

1 teaspoon toasted sesame oil

ITALIAN CAULI-RICE

2 tablespoons (30 ml) ghee or olive oil

2 tablespoons (8 g/0.3 oz) chopped Italian herbs such as thyme, parsley, oregano, basil, and/or rosemary, or 1–2 teaspoons dried herbs

1 teaspoon fresh lemon zest

½ teaspoon onion powder

¼ teaspoon garlic powder

⅓ cup (30 g/1.1 oz) grated Parmesan cheese

Salt and pepper, to taste

SOUTHWEST CAULI-RICE

2 tablespoons (30 ml) ghee or olive oil

1 teaspoon ground cumin

½ teaspoon onion powder

½ teaspoon smoked paprika

2 tablespoons (8 g/0.3 oz) chopped cilantro

2 tablespoons (30 ml) lime juice

⅛ teaspoon cayenne pepper

Salt and pepper, to taste

Run the cauliflower florets through a hand grater or food processor with a grating blade. Pulse until the florets resemble grains of rice.

FOR EGG FRIED CAULI-RICE: Heat a large saucepan greased with 1 tablespoon (15 ml) of ghee over medium-high heat. Crack the eggs into a mixing bowl, and season with a pinch of salt and pepper. Lightly whisk with a fork and pour into the hot pan. Cook for 1 to 2 minutes, or until scrambled, mixing it with a spatula. Once cooked, transfer to a plate and set aside.

Grease the pan with 2 tablespoons (30 ml) of ghee and add the white parts of the spring onions and the garlic. Cook for 1 minute, until fragrant. Add the cauli-rice and cook for 5 to 7 minutes, stirring constantly. Add the coconut aminos, stir, and take off the heat. Season with salt and pepper, add the green parts of the spring onions, the sesame oil, and the scrambled eggs. Stir to combine.

FOR ITALIAN OR SOUTHWEST CAULI-RICE: Grease a large saucepan with 2 tablespoons (30 ml) of ghee. Add all the aromatics apart from fresh herbs. Mix and cook over medium-low heat for up to 1 minute. Add the Parmesan (for Italian) and the cauli-rice and cook for 5 to 7 minutes, stirring constantly. Season with salt and pepper and add fresh herbs.

To store, let it cool and place in a sealed container. Refrigerate for up to 5 days.

TIP:

Make cauli-rice using just two to three ingredients! Just add Simple Pesto (page 16) with olive oil or ghee or try with harissa paste, chipotle chile paste, or Thai curry paste.

PICTURED ON PAGE 59

NUTRITION FACTS PER SERVING
(ABOUT 1 CUP EGG FRIED/ITALIAN/SOUTHWEST CAULI-RICE):
Total carbs: 8.4/9.8/10.2 g / Fiber: 3/3.8/3.9 g / Net carbs: 5.4/6/6.3 g / Protein: 6.7/6.3/3.7 g / Fat: 13.2/10/8.2 g / Calories: 173/145/119 kcal
Macronutrient ratio: Calories from carbs (13/17/22%), protein (16/18/13%), fat (71/65/65%)

Veggie Fritters Three Ways

SERVINGS: 5 (15 fritters total)
HANDS-ON TIME: 30 minutes
OVERALL TIME: 30 minutes

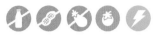

These veggie fritters are so good, and I simply couldn't share just one recipe! Here are my three favorite ways to make them. They're perfect for lunch boxes and on-the-go snacking.

3 medium (600 g/1.3 lb.) zucchini

8 ounces (227 g) frozen spinach, thawed and squeezed dry (weight excludes water squeezed out)

4 large eggs

½ teaspoon salt, or to taste

¼ teaspoon black pepper, or to taste

3 tablespoons (24 g/0.9 oz) coconut flour

¼ cup (60 ml) ghee, olive oil, or duck fat, divided

HERBY PARMESAN FRITTERS

1 tablespoon (3 g/0.1 oz) dried Italian herbs

½ teaspoon red pepper flakes

1 tablespoon (7 g/0.2 oz) onion powder

1 teaspoon garlic powder

⅓ cup (30 g/1.1 oz) grated Parmesan cheese

GOLDEN FRITTERS

1 tablespoon (6 g/0.2 oz) mild curry powder

½ teaspoon turmeric powder

1½ teaspoons onion powder

¾ teaspoon garlic powder

2 tablespoons (8 g/0.3 oz) chopped cilantro or parsley

SMOKY FRITTERS

1 tablespoon (7 g/0.2 oz) sweet paprika

1½ teaspoons onion powder

¾ teaspoon garlic powder

¾ teaspoon smoked paprika or ground chipotle chile

2 tablespoons (8 g/0.3 oz) chopped cilantro or parsley

Grate the zucchini and place in a bowl lined with cheesecloth. Twist the cheesecloth around the zucchini and squeeze out as much liquid as you can. You should end up with about 13 ounces (370 g) of drained zucchini.

In a mixing bowl, mix together the zucchini, spinach, eggs, salt, and pepper. Add the coconut flour and stir again. Add the remaining ingredients for the fritters you want to make: Herby Parmesan, Golden, or Smoky Fritters. Mix through.

Heat a large pan greased with 1 tablespoon (15 ml) of ghee over medium heat. Once hot, use a ¼-cup measuring cup to make the fritters (about 57 g/2 oz each). Shape with your hands and place in the hot pan. Cook them in batches for 3 to 4 minutes per side, until golden and crisp. Grease the pan between each batch until you use up all the ghee.

Eat warm or cold as a side or snack. Store in the fridge for up to 4 days or freeze for up to 3 months.

NUTRITION FACTS PER SERVING (3 HERBY PARMESAN/GOLDEN/SMOKY FRITTERS):
Total carbs: 9.8/9.2/9.2 g / Fiber: 4/4.3/4.1 g / Net carbs: 5.8/4.9/5.1 g / Protein: 11.5/9.4/9.4 g /
Fat: 18.9/17.4/17.4 g / Calories: 251/227/227 kcal
Macronutrient ratio: Calories from carbs (10/9/9%), protein (19/18/17%), fat (71/73/74%)

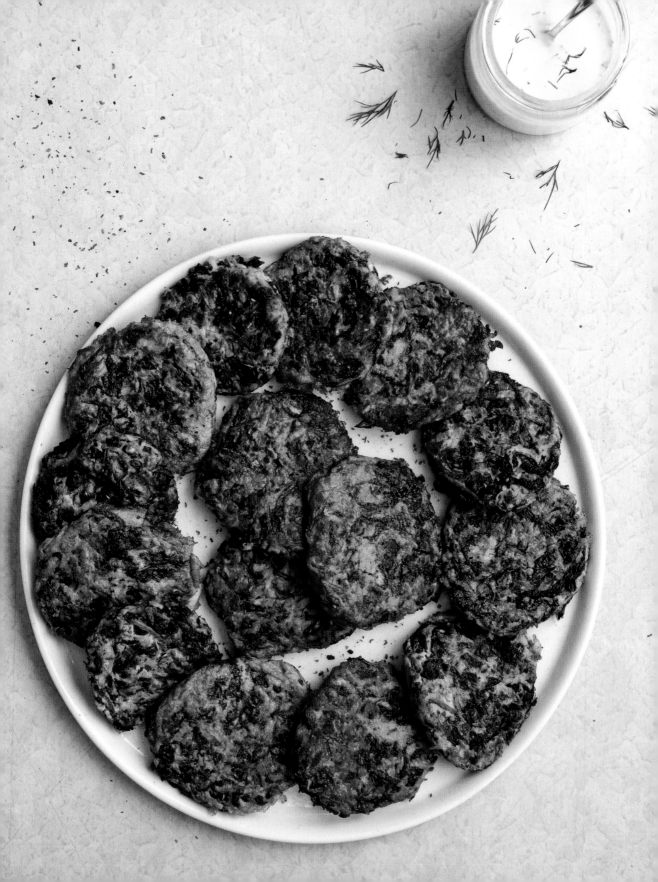

Cauli-Mash Three Ways

SERVINGS: 4
HANDS-ON TIME: 5 to 10 minutes
OVERALL TIME: 15 to 20 minutes

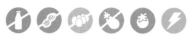

Cauli-mash is another keto staple that is really easy to prepare. You can always keep it basic by just using healthy fats, salt, and pepper. I prefer mine with a flavor boost from herbs and spices. If you're not sure which one to try first, go for the caramelized onion!

1 medium (600 g/1.3 lb.) cauliflower

½ teaspoon salt, or to taste

¼ teaspoon black pepper, or to taste

CARAMELIZED ONION CAULI-MASH

¼ cup (60 ml) ghee, butter, or extra-virgin olive oil

1 small (70 g/2.5 oz) yellow onion, chopped

1 clove garlic, minced

2 tablespoons (8 g/0.3 oz) chopped herbs or 1–2 teaspoons dried herbs of choice (parsley, rosemary, and thyme work best)

SOUR CREAM & DILL CAULI-MASH

½ cup (115 g/4.1 oz) sour cream

2 tablespoons (8 g/0.3 oz) chopped dill or 2 teaspoons (2 g/0.1 oz) dried dill

1 teaspoon onion powder

CHEESY CAULI-MASH

½ cup (120 g/4.2 oz) full-fat cream cheese

½ cup (57 g/2 oz) grated Cheddar cheese

Cut the cauliflower into medium-size florets and place them in a steamer. Cook for about 10 minutes. Remove from the heat and place in a blender.

TO MAKE THE CARAMELIZED ONION CAULI-MASH: Grease a pan with 2 tablespoons (30 ml) of ghee and add the onion. Cook for 5 to 7 minutes, or until golden brown. Add the garlic and cook for 1 minute. Take off the heat. Add it to the blender (optionally leaving some onion for topping) together with the steamed cauliflower and remaining 2 tablespoons (30 ml) ghee and process until smooth and creamy. Season to taste.

TO MAKE THE SOUR CREAM & DILL OR CHEESY CAULI-MASH: To the blender with the cauliflower, add the remaining ingredients. Process until smooth and creamy. Optionally, you can leave some Cheddar, herbs, or ghee for garnish.

Serve immediately, or let it cool down and store in a sealed container in the fridge for up to 4 days.

TIP:

If you like the flavor of caramelized cauliflower (yum!), instead of steaming the cauliflower, bake the florets in the oven at 400°F (200°C) forced fan or 425°F (220°C) conventional for 10 minutes covered with parchment paper, and then another 20 minutes with the parchment removed. Then blend just like you would with steamed cauliflower.

PICTURED ON PAGE 59

NUTRITION FACTS PER SERVING (ABOUT 1 CUP CARAMELIZED ONION/SOUR CREAM & DILL/CHEESY CAULI-MASH):
Total carbs: 9.4/9.4/9 g / Fiber: 3.5/3.1/3.1 g / Net carbs: 5.9/6.3/5.9 g / Protein: 3.2/3.7/8.2 g /
Fat: 14.2/19.8/27.3 g / Calories: 171/222/293 kcal
Macronutrient ratio: Calories from carbs (14/12/8%), protein (8/7/11%), fat (78/81/81%)

Three-Minute Keto Bread, Three Ways

SERVINGS: 2
HANDS-ON TIME: 5 minutes
OVERALL TIME: 10 minutes

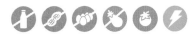

Most keto bread recipes take hours to prepare, but this one is done in less than ten minutes with only three minutes to cook. I included three recipes so that everyone can make a quick and easy keto bread no matter what your dietary restrictions are!

BASIC KETO BREAD

¼ cup (25 g/0.8 oz) almond flour

¼ cup (28 g/1 oz) flax meal

2 teaspoons (5 g/0.2 oz) psyllium husk powder

¼ teaspoon gluten-free baking powder

Pinch of salt and pepper

1 large egg

¼ cup (60 ml) water

CHEESY KETO BREAD

¼ cup (25 g/0.8 oz) almond flour

⅓ cup (30 g/1.1 oz) grated Parmesan cheese

2 teaspoons (5 g/0.2 oz) psyllium husk powder

¼ teaspoon gluten-free baking powder

Pinch of salt and pepper

1 large egg

2 tablespoons (30 ml) water

ALLERGY-FREE KETO BREAD

2 tablespoons (16 g/0.6 oz) coconut flour

¼ cup (28 g/1 oz) flax meal

2 teaspoons (5 g/0.2 oz) psyllium husk powder

Pinch of salt and pepper

½ teaspoon gluten-free baking powder

½ cup (120 ml) water

In one bowl, mix all the dry ingredients for the recipe you want to make. In another bowl, mix the wet ingredients. Combine the two and then set aside for 5 minutes.

Divide between two ramekins and microwave on high for 2 to 3 minutes, checking every 30 to 60 seconds to avoid overcooking. If the bread ends up too dry, you can "rehydrate" it by evenly pouring a tablespoon (15 ml) of water on top of it, then return it to the microwave for another 30 seconds.

Store at room temperature in a sealed container for 1 day, in the fridge for up to 5 days, or freeze for up to 3 months.

TIP:

If you don't have a microwave, you can make these in the oven set to 350°F (175°C) forced fan or 380°F (195°C) conventional and bake for about 15 minutes.

PICTURED ON PAGE 59

NUTRITION FACTS PER SERVING (BASIC/CHEESY/ALLERGY-FREE KETO BREAD):
Total carbs: 8.7/5.2/8.6 g / Fiber: 6.8/3.1/7 g / Net carbs: 1.9/2.1/1.6 g / Protein: 8.5/11.3/4 g / Fat: 14.9/12.8/7.1 g / Calories: 186/170/107 kcal Macronutrient ratio: Calories from carbs (4/5/7%), protein (19/27/19%), fat (77/68/74%)

Zucchini Gratin

SERVINGS: 8
HANDS-ON TIME: 15 minutes
OVERALL TIME: 50 minutes

Baked zucchini in creamy cheese sauce with no thickeners and no potatoes! This is also easy to scale up or down and so you can even serve it as a main dish. For extra protein, add some crisp bacon or cooked chicken.

½ cup (120 ml) heavy whipping cream

¼ cup (57 g/2 oz) unsalted butter

1 cup (240 g/8.5 oz) cream cheese

½ teaspoon onion powder

½ teaspoon garlic powder

2 cups (227 g/8 oz) grated Cheddar cheese, divided

¼ cup (15 g/0.5 oz) chopped herbs such as parsley, thyme, and chives, or 2–3 teaspoons (2–3 g) dried Italian herbs

Salt and pepper, to taste

4 medium (800 g/1.8 lb.) zucchini

Place the cream and butter in a small saucepan and gently heat it up. Add the cream cheese, stir until melted, and bring to a simmer. Once you see bubbles, take it off the heat. Add the onion powder, garlic powder, and 1 cup (113 g/4 oz) of Cheddar and mix until smooth and creamy. Stir in the herbs. Taste and season if needed.

Preheat the oven to 340°F (170°C) forced fan or 375°F (190°C) conventional. Cut the zucchini into about ½-inch (1 cm) thick round slices.

Place a layer of zucchini in a baking dish large enough for the zucchini and about 2 cups (480 ml) of cheese sauce. Pour some of the cheese sauce over the zucchini and repeat for the remaining zucchini and cheese sauce. Finally, sprinkle the top with the remaining 1 cup (113 g/4 oz) of Cheddar cheese.

Bake for 35 to 40 minutes, or until bubbly and golden on top. Serve warm, or let it cool down and refrigerate for up to 5 days.

TIP:

Apart from adding different herbs and spices, you can use different types of cheese. Try swapping cream cheese for soft goat's cheese, or grated Cheddar for Swiss cheese or sheep's cheese.

NUTRITION FACTS PER SERVING:
Total carbs: 5.3 g / Fiber: 1.2 g / Net carbs: 4.1 g / Protein: 9.2 g / Fat: 25.4 g / Calories: 276 kcal
Macronutrient ratio: Calories from carbs (6%), protein (13%), fat (81%

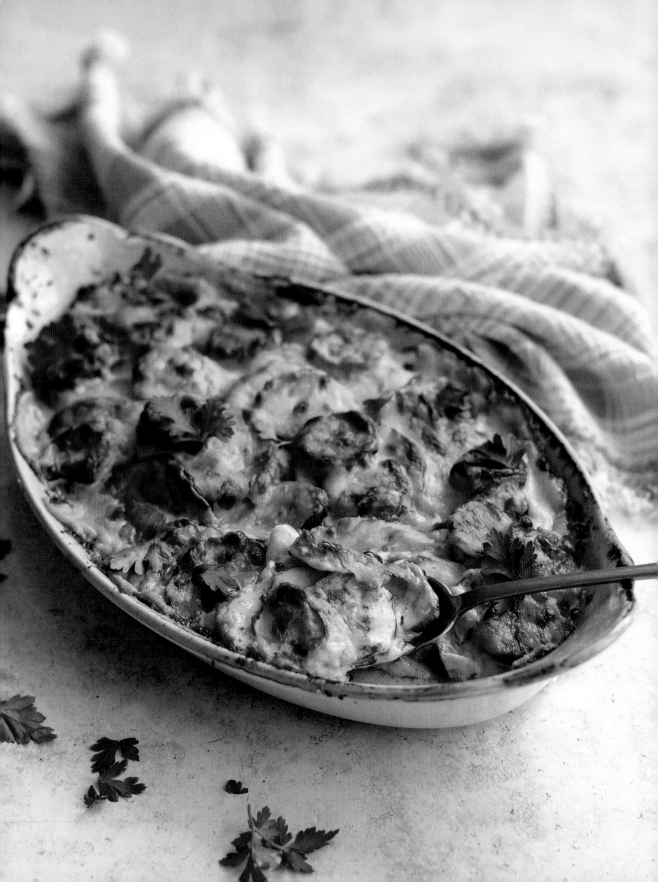

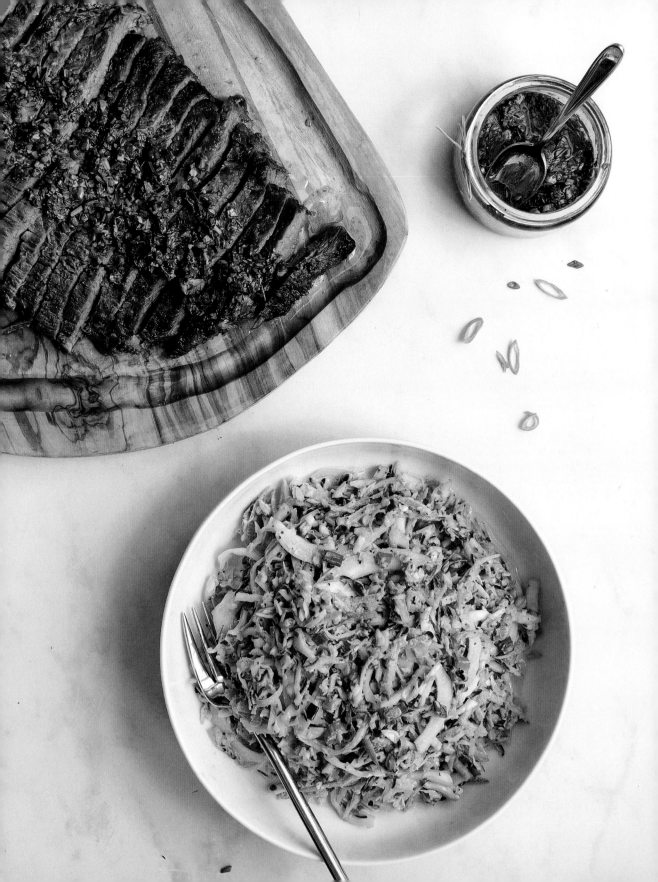

Pink Coleslaw

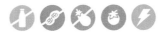

SERVINGS: 4
HANDS-ON TIME: 15 minutes
OVERALL TIME: 45 minutes

Coleslaw is the perfect side for pulled pork or any grilled meat. I used more red cabbage to give the coleslaw its beautiful pink hue and to boost the nutritional values, as red cabbage contains more antioxidants and vitamins than green cabbage. You can easily double the batch!

DRESSING

6 tablespoons (90/3.2 oz) mayonnaise
    (page 16)
1 tablespoon (15 ml) apple cider
    vinegar
1 tablespoon (15 ml) fresh lemon juice
Salt and pepper, to taste
Optional: 1 tablespoon (10 g/0.4 oz)
    powdered erythritol or Swerve
1 medium (15 g/0.5 oz) spring onion,
    sliced

COLESLAW MIX

2½ cups (175 g/6.2 oz) shredded green
    or white cabbage
1½ cups (105 g/3.7 oz) shredded red
    cabbage
1 small (57 g/2 oz) carrot, shredded

TO MAKE THE DRESSING: In a small bowl, mix the mayo, vinegar, lemon juice, salt, and pepper. Optionally mix in erythritol. Mix in the sliced spring onion and optionally reserve some for topping.

TO MAKE THE COLESLAW: Prepare the coleslaw mix by placing the cabbage and carrot in a large mixing bowl. Pour the dressing over the veggies and toss to combine. Cover and refrigerate for 30 to 60 minutes before serving. Store in the fridge in a sealed container for up to 4 days.

TIPS:

• Short on time? Use ready-made coleslaw mix made with cabbage and carrots. Avoid products that already include dressing.
• Have any leftover broccoli stalks? Peel and slice them and add them to the salad instead of part of the green cabbage!
• Optionally, you can add 2 to 3 teaspoons (12 to 18 g/0.4 to 0.7 oz) of whole-grain mustard and/or ½ teaspoon of dried celery seeds.

NUTRITION FACTS PER SERVING (ABOUT 1 CUP/115 G/4 OZ):
Total carbs: 6.6 g / Fiber: 2.3 g / Net carbs: 4.3 g / Protein: 1.3 g / Fat: 18.8 g / Calories: 193 kcal
Macronutrient ratio: Calories from carbs (9%), protein (3%), fat (88%)

Chapter 5
Soups & Salads

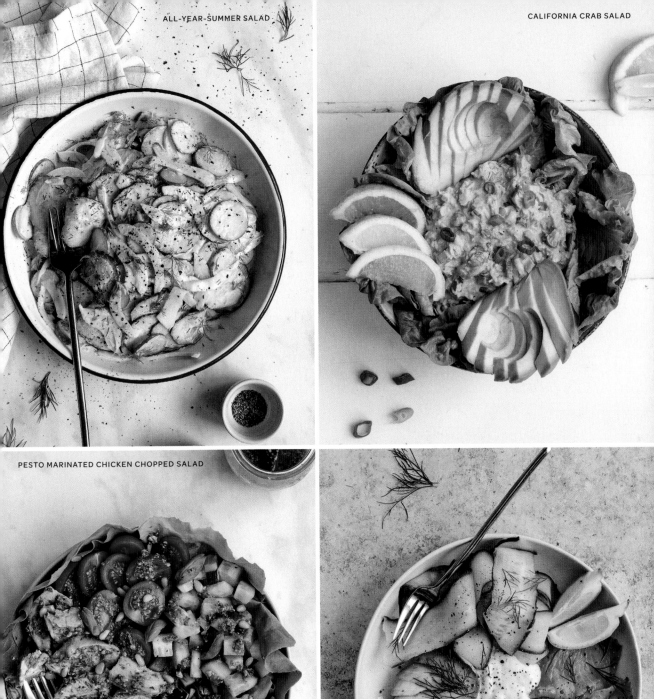

ALL-YEAR-SUMMER SALAD

CALIFORNIA CRAB SALAD

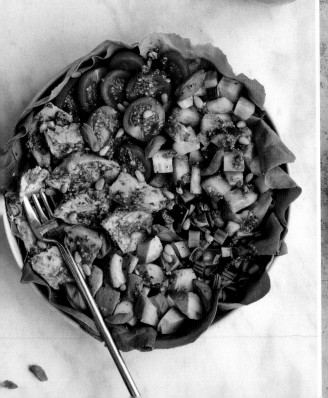

PESTO MARINATED CHICKEN CHOPPED SALAD

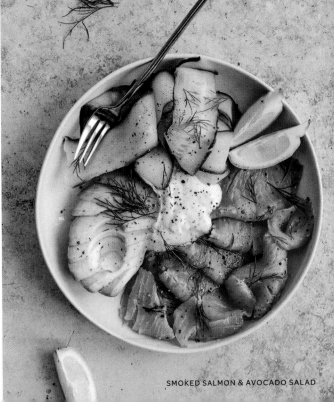

SMOKED SALMON & AVOCADO SALAD

Oyster Mushroom Soup

SERVINGS: 6
HANDS-ON TIME: 10 minutes
OVERALL TIME: 30 minutes

Thick and creamy soups and stews are an essential part of Czech cuisine. When I was a kid, my mom used to make this delicious recipe adapted from beef tripe (cow stomach) soup. It's similar to goulash, with strong flavor from paprika, marjoram, onion, and garlic. Sometimes she swapped tripe for oyster mushrooms because they were easier to find. I swapped potatoes for cauliflower and part-blended the soup to get an ultra-rich and creamy result, no potatoes and no flour needed!

¼ cup (60 ml) ghee, duck fat, or lard

1 medium (110 g/3.9 oz) yellow onion, chopped

1 pound (450 g) oyster mushrooms, sliced

1½ tablespoons (10 g/0.4 oz) sweet paprika

5 cups (1.2 L) beef stock or vegetable stock

½ small (250 g/8.8 oz) cauliflower, cut into small florets

1 teaspoon marjoram, or to taste

2 cloves garlic, crushed

Heat a large pot greased with ghee over medium-high heat. Add the onion and cook for 5 minutes, until lightly golden. Add the mushrooms and cook for 5 minutes. Add the paprika, stock, and cauliflower. Bring to a boil, reduce the heat to low, and cover with a lid. Cook for 8 to 10 minutes, until the cauliflower is tender.

Ladle about half of the soup into a blender or use an immersion blender. Process until smooth and creamy. Return the soup to the pot and add the marjoram and garlic. Mix to combine. Season to taste and serve hot, or let it cool down and refrigerate for up to 5 days. Serve on its own or with some sour cream and Three-Minute Keto Bread (page 67).

TIP:

You can easily convert this into a satisfying stew by reducing the amount of stock and adding fatty protein (such as pork belly or pork shoulder). Cook it over low heat with the lid on for 60 to 90 minutes, or until tender.

NUTRITION FACTS PER SERVING (ABOUT 1½ CUPS/360 ML):
Total carbs: 9.9 g / Fiber: 3.6 g / Net carbs: 6.3 g / Protein: 6.8 g / Fat: 13.2 g / Calories: 172 kcal
Macronutrient ratio: Calories from carbs (15%), protein (16%), fat (69%)

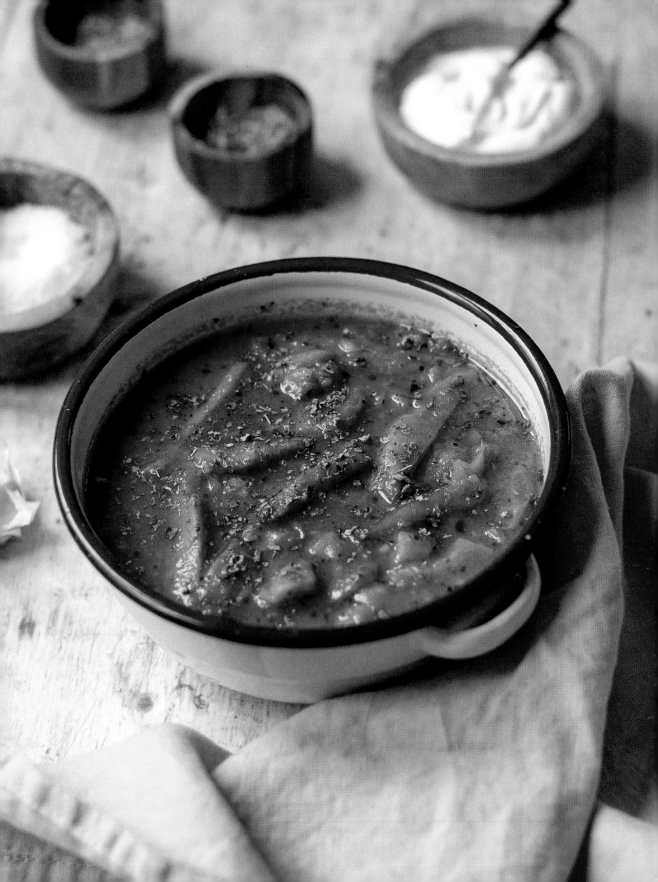

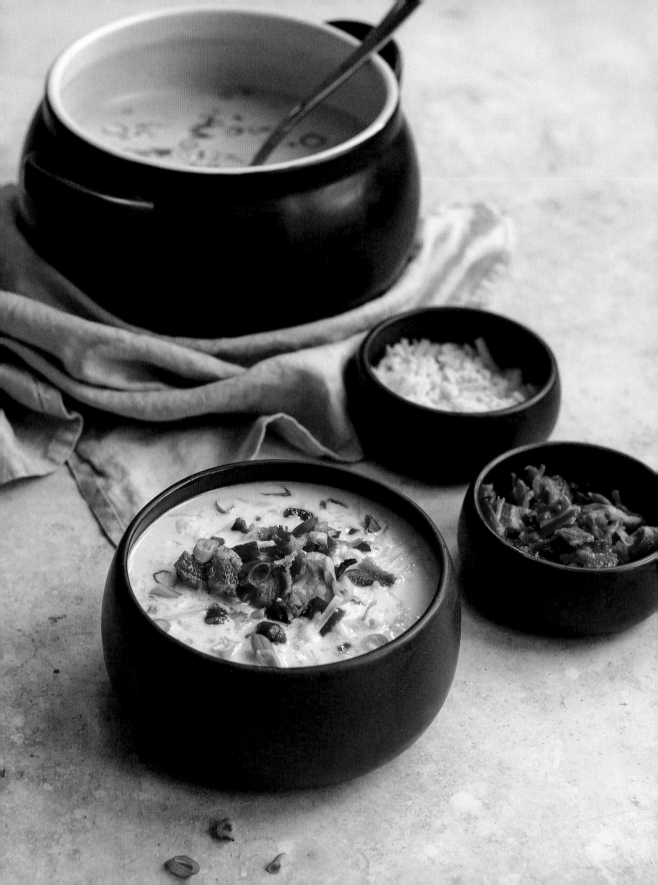

Loaded Notato Soup

SERVINGS: 6
HANDS-ON TIME: 15 minutes
OVERALL TIME: 30 minutes

This creamy soup is the ultimate comfort food! It's a great one-pot meal that doesn't require too much preparation. Serve with cheese and crispy bacon on top, and some keto bread (page 67).

2 tablespoons (30 ml) ghee, duck fat, or lard, divided

1 small (70 g/2.5 oz) yellow onion, diced

2 cloves garlic, minced

1 small (450 g/1 lb.) cauliflower, chopped

4 cups (960 ml) beef or chicken stock

¾ cup (180 ml) heavy whipping cream

¾ cup (170 g/6 oz) sour cream

1½ cups (170 g/6 oz) shredded Cheddar cheese, divided

3 medium (45 g/1.5 oz) spring onions, sliced

Salt and pepper, to taste

6 slices (96 g/3.4 oz) crispy bacon (see page 14), crumbled

Heat a large pot greased with ghee over medium-high heat. Add the onion and cook for 5 minutes, until lightly golden. Add the garlic and cauliflower and cook for 1 minute. Pour in the stock and bring to a boil. Reduce the heat to low and cover with a lid. Cook for 8 to 10 minutes, until the cauliflower is tender. Add the cream and sour cream. Heat through and then take off the heat.

Ladle about half of the soup with 1 cup (113 g/4 oz) of the Cheddar into a blender or use an immersion blender. Process until smooth and creamy. Pour back into the pot and add half of the spring onions. Season with salt and pepper. Serve with crispy bacon pieces, the remaining ½ cup (56 g/2 oz) Cheddar cheese, and the remaining spring onions. Once cooled, store in a sealed jar in the fridge for up to 4 days.

NUTRITION FACTS PER SERVING (1½ CUPS/360 ML):
Total carbs: 8.9 g / Fiber: 2 g / Net carbs: 6.9 g / Protein: 16.7 g / Fat: 35.2 g / Calories: 413 kcal
Macronutrient ratio: Calories from carbs (7%), protein (16%), fat (77%)

Pesto Egg Drop Soup

SERVINGS: 6
HANDS-ON TIME: 10 minutes
OVERALL TIME: 20 minutes

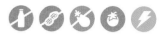

This is my go-to soup for those days I barely find ten minutes to cook. Using pesto works in two ways; it adds a fantastic flavor boost and it's a great source of healthy fats! The basic recipe only uses kale, but feel free to add your favorite veggies, grated Parmesan, or even cooked chicken.

2 quarts (2 L) chicken stock or vegetable stock

¾ pound (340 g) dark-leaf Italian kale or greens of choice (curly kale, chard, collards, savoy cabbage, or spinach)

4 large eggs

6 tablespoons (90 g/3.2 oz) pesto (page 16)

Salt and pepper, to taste

Optional add-ons: cooked chicken, sliced mushrooms, grated Parmesan cheese, and/or more veggies such as broccoli, cauliflower, and carrots

Pour the stock into a large pot and heat over medium heat, until it starts to simmer. If you are using any add-on veggies that require a longer cooking time, add them now and cook until tender. Add the kale and cook for 1 to 3 minutes, until tender.

In a bowl, whisk the eggs with pesto and slowly pour them into the simmering soup. Keep stirring until the egg is cooked and then take off the heat. Season with salt and pepper. Pour into a serving bowl.

Eat immediately, or let it cool down and store in a sealed container for up to 5 days.

TIP:

I make my chicken stock in an electric pressure cooker. Simply place a whole chicken in the electric pressure cooker and add water until about three-quarters full. Close the lid and seal. Press "Poultry" or set to cook on high pressure for 45 minutes. In less than an hour you'll have stock and the deliciously tender chicken.

NUTRITION FACTS PER SERVING (2 CUPS/480 ML):
Total carbs: 4.2 g / Fiber: 2.2 g / Net carbs: 2 g / Protein: 9.2 g / Fat: 16.2 g / Calories: 188 kcal
Macronutrient ratio: Calories from carbs (4%), protein (19%), fat (77%)

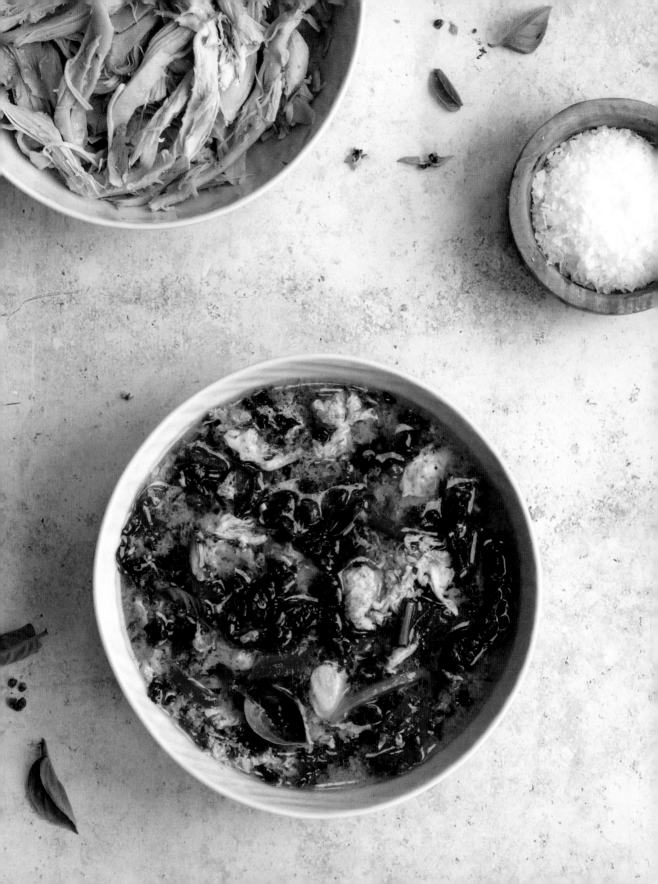

All-Year-Summer Salad

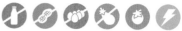

SERVINGS: 6
HANDS-ON TIME: 10 minutes
OVERALL TIME: 10 minutes

This easy salad always reminds me of a warm summer day. It's based on a classic cucumber salad with additional radishes and fennel, which pair really well with the other ingredients. You can eat it as a light dish or as a side, and it's great for barbecues, too.

1 bulb (200 g/7.1 oz) fennel
6 large (140 g/5 oz) radishes
1 large (350 g/12.4 oz) cucumber

DRESSING
½ cup (115 g/4.1 oz) sour cream
2 tablespoons (30 ml) extra-virgin olive oil
1 clove garlic, crushed
1 teaspoon fresh lemon zest
1 tablespoon (15 ml) fresh lemon juice
1 teaspoon Dijon mustard
½ teaspoon onion powder
2 tablespoons (8 g/0.3 oz) reserved chopped fennel fronds or dill, plus more for garnish
Salt and pepper, to taste

If there are any fronds on the fennel bulb, reserve them for the dressing and garnish. Thinly slice the fennel, radishes, and cucumber. Alternatively, use a slicing blade on your food processor. Place in a large mixing bowl.

TO MAKE THE DRESSING: Mix all the remaining ingredients in a small bowl. Add the dressing to the sliced vegetables and mix to combine. If you have time, place in the fridge for 30 to 60 minutes to allow the flavors to combine. Store in the fridge for up to 3 days. The veggies will release their juices, so the salad is always best eaten fresh.

TIP:
Are you dairy-free? Swap the sour cream for mayonnaise (page 16)!

PICTURED ON PAGE 73

NUTRITION FACTS PER SERVING:
Total carbs: 6.1 g / Fiber: 2 g / Net carbs: 4.1 g / Protein: 1.5 g / Fat: 8.4 g / Calories: 102 kcal
Macronutrient ratio: Calories from carbs (17%), protein (6%), fat (77%)

California Crab Salad

SERVINGS: 2
HANDS-ON TIME: 10 minutes
OVERALL TIME: 10 minutes

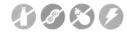

Let's be real, travel is often about food! I was fortunate to try some of the best dishes during my recent U.S. travels. Crab salad ended up being my absolute favorite meal during the entire trip! It's such a refreshing and satisfying salad that always reminds me of the beautiful beaches in California. And it's naturally low in carbs, packed with flavor, protein, and healthy fats.

CREAMY CRAB

⅓ cup (73 g/2.6 oz) mayonnaise (page 16)

½ teaspoon fresh lemon zest

1 tablespoon (15 ml) fresh lemon or lime juice

1 tablespoon (15 ml) sriracha sauce (for hot) or tomato paste (for mild)

1 tablespoon (4 g/0.2 oz) chopped dill or 1 teaspoon dried dill

1 clove garlic, crushed

7 ounces (200 g) cooked crabmeat

2 medium (70 g/2.5 oz) celery sticks, sliced

2 medium (30 g/1.1 oz) spring onions, chopped

Salt and pepper, to taste

SALAD

1 small head (200 g/7.1 oz) green lettuce (romaine, butter, or gem)

2 small (200 g/7.1 oz) avocados, sliced

Optional: lemon wedges

TO MAKE THE CRAB: In a bowl, combine the mayo, lemon zest, lemon juice, sriracha sauce, dill, and garlic. Mix to combine and add the crab, celery, and spring onions. You can reserve some spring onions for garnish. Season with salt and pepper.

TO ASSEMBLE THE SALAD: Place the lettuce leaves into two bowls. Top each with the creamy crab filling, avocado, and optionally serve with lemon wedges. The crab filling can be stored in the fridge for up to 3 days.

TIPS:

• You can use fresh cooked crabmeat or canned crabmeat. Alternatively, use cooked and chopped shrimp. Optionally, you can add a pinch of Old Bay seasoning.

• Instead of regular salad, you can make these as stuffed avocados! Simply omit the lettuce, scoop the middle of the avocado out, leaving ½ inch (1 cm) of the avocado flesh. Cut the scooped avocado into small pieces and add it to the crab. Fill each avocado half with the crab and avocado mixture.

• This recipe also makes a great portable lunch option. Simply place the creamy crab filling in a wide-mouth jar, followed by diced avocado and chopped lettuce or any greens, and seal with a lid. Shake just before serving and eat from the jar or transfer to a plate.

PICTURED ON PAGE 73

NUTRITION FACTS PER SERVING:
Total carbs: 16 g / Fiber: 9.4 g / Net carbs: 6.6 g / Protein: 23.7 g / Fat: 47.8 g / Calories: 568 kcal
Macronutrient ratio: Calories from carbs (5%), protein (17%), fat (78%)

The Easiest Fish Salad

SERVINGS: 2
HANDS-ON TIME: 5 to 10 minutes
OVERALL TIME: 5 to 10 minutes

This is my go-to keto meal for ultra-busy days. It takes very few steps, ingredients, and prep time, but gives maximum nutrients, healthy fats, and protein. Sometimes I swap the tuna for salmon, mackerel, or sardines. Sometimes I add sliced avocado for extra fats or hard-boiled egg for extra protein.

⅓ cup (73 g/2.6 oz) mayonnaise (page 16)
½ teaspoon Dijon mustard
1 teaspoon fresh lemon juice
Salt and pepper, to taste
1 small head (200 g/7.1 oz) green lettuce (romaine, butter, or gem)
1 cup (10 g/0.4 oz) arugula or watercress
½ small (30 g/1.1 oz) red onion, sliced
½ medium (140 g/5 oz) cucumber, sliced
10 small (113 g/4 oz) cherry tomatoes, halved
7 ounces (200 g) drained canned tuna, flaked
12 whole (28 g/1 oz) pitted olives
Optional: 1 medium (150 g/5.3 oz) sliced avocado or hard-boiled egg

In a small bowl, mix the mayo with the Dijon mustard and lemon juice. Season with salt and pepper.

TO ASSEMBLE THE SALAD: Place the lettuce leaves into two bowls. Top each with arugula, onion, cucumber, tomatoes, tuna, and olives. Optionally, you can add avocado or hard-boiled egg. Drizzle with the prepared dressing and serve.

To store, refrigerate for up to 1 day.

TIPS:
- Swap the tuna for any canned fish such as sardines, mackerel, salmon, or herring.
- Are you egg-free? Instead of mayo, you can use a simple Italian vinaigrette made with ¼ cup (60 ml) extra-virgin olive oil, 1 tablespoon (15 ml) fresh lemon juice, ½ teaspoon balsamic vinegar, 1 tablespoon (4 g/0.2 oz) chopped oregano, basil, and/or thyme (or 1 teaspoon dried herbs), ½ teaspoon Dijon or whole-grain mustard, salt, and pepper.

NUTRITION FACTS PER SERVING:
Total carbs: 8.6 g / Fiber: 3.4 g / Net carbs: 5.2 g / Protein: 25.3 g / Fat: 35.8 g / Calories: 448 kcal
Macronutrient ratio: Calories from carbs (5%), protein (23%), fat (72%)

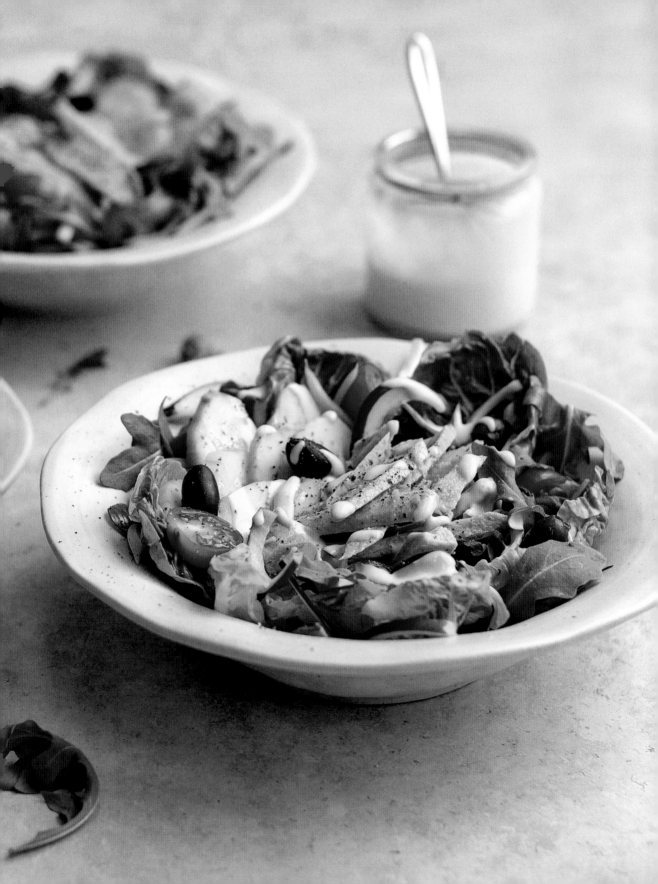

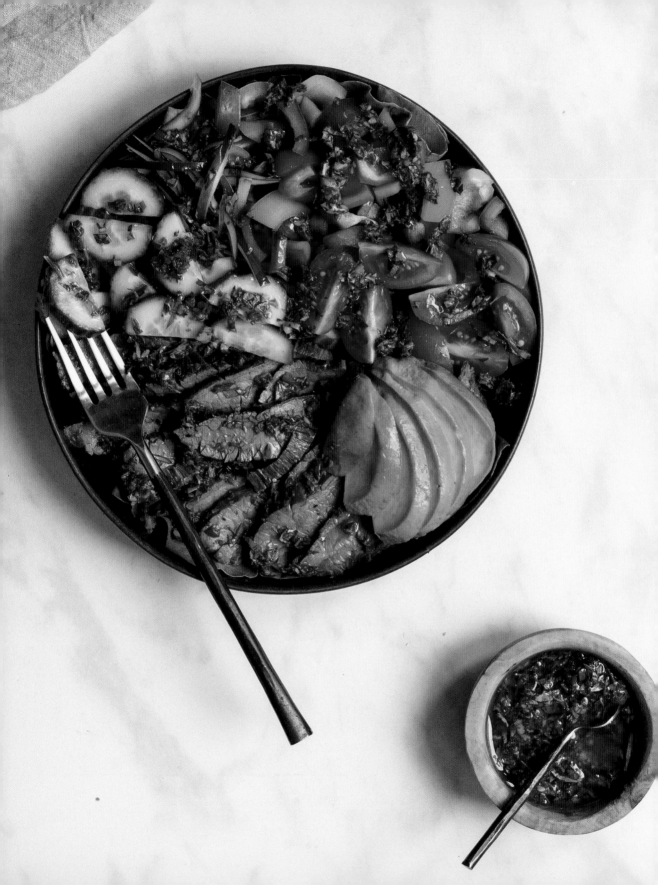

Chimichurri Steak Salad Bowl

SERVINGS: 2
HANDS-ON TIME: 10 minutes
OVERALL TIME: 15 minutes

Chimichurri is on my list of the best ever condiments. It's always the first item I look for on the menu in a steak bar! I love this salad because it's ridiculously easy and it's also a great way to use leftover steak or even cooked chicken.

SALAD

1 large (340 g/12 oz) flank steak or skirt steak

Pinch of salt and pepper

1–2 teaspoons ghee, duck fat, or olive oil, for frying

6– 8 leaves (100 g/3.5 oz) green lettuce (romaine, butter, or gem)

½ small (85 g/3 oz) cucumber, sliced

½ small (30 g/1.1 oz) red onion, sliced

1 small (100 g/3.5 oz) avocado, sliced

8 small (100 g/3.5 oz) cherry tomatoes, halved

1 cup (113 g/4 oz) roughly chopped mixed bell peppers

¼ cup (60 ml) chimichurri (recipe below)

CHIMICHURRI

1 large (60 g/2.1 oz) bunch fresh parsley

¼ cup (15 g/0.5 oz) chopped fresh oregano

4 cloves garlic, chopped

1 small (5 g/0.2 oz) red chile pepper, seeds removed

2 tablespoons (30 ml) apple cider vinegar or fresh lime juice

½ cup (120 ml) extra-virgin olive oil

Salt and pepper, to taste

TO COOK THE STEAK: Pat dry the steak and season with salt and pepper. Set a large pan greased with the ghee over high heat. Once hot, cook the steak for 3 minutes on each side (flank steak), or 2 to 3 minutes on each side (skirt steak), depending on the thickness of the meat, until medium-rare. Do not overcook the steak. Remove from the pan and keep warm. Slice when ready to serve.

TO MAKE THE CHIMICHURRI: For chunky chimichurri, finely chop the ingredients. For a smooth sauce, place all the ingredients in a blender and process until smooth. Season to taste. Store any leftover chimichurri in a sealed jar in the fridge for 1 to 2 weeks.

TO ASSEMBLE THE SALAD: Place the lettuce leaves in serving bowls and add the sliced steak, cucumber, onion, avocado, tomatoes, and bell peppers. You can mix or keep all ingredients separate. Drizzle each bowl with 3 tablespoons (45 ml) of chimichurri.

NUTRITION FACTS PER SERVING:
Total carbs: 15.9 g / Fiber: 7.6 g / Net carbs: 8.3 g / Protein: 39.6 g / Fat: 43.4 g / Calories: 609 kcal
Macronutrient ratio: Calories from carbs (6%), protein (27%), fat (67%)

Pesto Marinated Chicken Chopped Salad

SERVINGS: 2
HANDS-ON TIME: 10 minutes
OVERALL TIME: 30 minutes

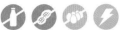

This simple lunch box dish proves that salads are so much more than just a bunch of greens with dressing. Juicy chicken slices marinated in pesto and served with creamy avocado and crispy veggies—what's not to love? You can also swap the chicken for sliced steak, pork tenderloin, and even flaked salmon.

MARINATED CHICKEN

¼ cup (60 g/2.1 oz) pesto (page 16)
2 tablespoons (30 ml) extra-virgin
  olive oil
1 tablespoon (15 ml) fresh lemon juice
Salt and pepper, to taste
2 small (250 g/8.5 oz) cooked chicken
  breasts (poached or baked), sliced

SALAD

6–8 leaves (100 g/3.5 oz) green lettuce
  (romaine, butter, or gem)
½ small (30 g/1.1 oz) red onion, sliced
10 small (113 g/4 oz) cherry tomatoes,
  halved
½ medium (113 g/4 oz) cucumber,
  chopped
1 small (100 g/3.5 oz) avocado, diced
Optional: pine nuts and basil leaves

TO MAKE THE CHICKEN: Mix the pesto, olive oil, lemon juice, salt, and pepper in a bowl. Reserve about 2 tablespoons (30 ml) for later and use the rest for marinating the chicken. Place the chicken slices in a bowl and pour over the marinade, making sure that all the slices are covered. Place in the fridge for at least 20 minutes or overnight.

TO ASSEMBLE THE SALAD: Place the lettuce leaves in serving bowls. Add the sliced chicken, onion, tomatoes, cucumber, and avocado. Drizzle the veggies with the remaining marinade. Optionally, sprinkle with pine nuts and basil leaves.

The salad is best eaten fresh but can be refrigerated for up to 1 day. The marinated chicken can be stored in a sealed jar in the fridge for up to 4 days.

PICTURED ON PAGE 73

NUTRITION FACTS PER SERVING:
Total carbs: 12.1 g / Fiber: 6 g / Net carbs: 6.1 g / Protein: 39.8 g / Fat: 44.8 g / Calories: 603 kcal
Macronutrient ratio: Calories from carbs (4%), protein (27%), fat (69%)

Smoked Salmon & Avocado Salad

SERVINGS: 1
HANDS-ON TIME: 5 minutes
OVERALL TIME: 5 minutes

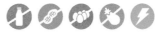

This single-serve salad bowl is packed with flavor from horseradish and smoked salmon. If you are thinking about eating salad for breakfast, this is the dish to go for!

DRESSING

2 tablespoons (30 g/1.1 oz)
  mayonnaise (page 16)
½ teaspoon prepared or fresh
  horseradish
1 teaspoon fresh lemon juice
Salt and pepper, to taste

SALAD

3½ ounces (100 g) smoked salmon
½ medium (75 g/2.7 oz) avocado,
  sliced
½ small (85 g/3 oz) cucumber,
  chopped or sliced into thin ribbons
1 teaspoon extra-virgin olive oil
A few sprigs of dill or herbs of choice
Salt and pepper, to taste
Lemon wedges

TO MAKE THE DRESSING: Mix the mayo, horseradish, lemon juice, salt, and pepper in a small bowl.

TO MAKE THE SALAD: Place the smoked salmon in a bowl and add the sliced avocado, cucumber, and dressing. Drizzle with the olive oil, sprinkle with dill, and season with salt and pepper. Serve immediately with lemon wedges.

TIP:

Are you egg-free? Swap the mayo for full-fat sour cream or crème fraîche.

PICTURED ON PAGE 73

NUTRITION FACTS PER SERVING:
Total carbs: 9.4 g / Fiber: 5.8 g / Net carbs: 3.6 g / Protein: 20.7 g / Fat: 44.9 g / Calories: 513 kcal
Macronutrient ratio: Calories from carbs (3%), protein (17%), fat (80%)

Grilled Ranch Chicken Salad Bowl

SERVINGS: 2
HANDS-ON TIME: 20 minutes
OVERALL TIME: 30 minutes

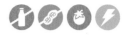

This is a great American-style salad with crispy chicken, bacon, and ranch dressing. It features grilled chicken breast, but you could even use skin-on crispy chicken thigh or steak. The great thing about low-carb diets being so popular is that there are more and more keto-friendly products, like ranch dressing, that are both low in carbs and use "clean" ingredients.

1 tablespoon (15 ml) ghee or duck fat

4 slices (120 g/4.2 oz) bacon

1 medium (200 g/7.1 oz) chicken breast

Pinch of salt and pepper

6–8 leaves (100 g/3.5 oz) green lettuce (romaine, butter, or gem)

4 large (100 g/3.5 oz) radishes, sliced

½ medium (113 g/4 oz) cucumber, chopped

8 small (100 g/3.5 oz) cherry tomatoes, halved or quartered

½ medium (57 g/2 oz) green bell pepper, sliced

¼ cup (60 ml) ranch dressing (see tip)

1 medium (15 g/0.5 oz) spring onion, chopped

1 large hard-boiled egg, quartered (see page 15)

Heat a griddle pan or a regular pan greased with ghee over medium-high heat. Add the bacon slices and cook until crispy. Remove from the pan, cut in half, and set aside. To the same pan, add the chicken breast and cook for 5 to 7 minutes per side. The internal temperature should read 165°F (75°C). Season with salt and pepper.

TO ASSEMBLE THE SALAD: Place the lettuce leaves in serving bowls and add the sliced grilled chicken, radishes, cucumber, tomatoes, and bell pepper. Add the bacon slices. Drizzle with the ranch dressing (2 tablespoons/30 ml per serving) and sprinkle with the spring onion. Top with the egg quarters. Season to taste.

TIP:

There are some good low-carb ranch dressing products you can buy (Primal Kitchen Ranch is also dairy-free). Instead of buying ready-made, you can make your own ranch dressing by mixing ¼ cup (55 g/1.9 oz) mayonnaise (page 16), ¼ cup (58 g/2 oz) sour cream, 1 tablespoon (15 ml) apple cider vinegar or fresh lemon juice, ¼ teaspoon onion powder, ¼ teaspoon garlic powder, ⅛ teaspoon paprika, and 1 tablespoon (4 g/0.2 oz) chopped herbs such as dill, parsley, and/or chives (or 1 teaspoon dried herbs). This will yield about ½ cup (120 ml). It's easy to scale up too! Store in a sealed jar in the fridge for up to 5 days.

NUTRITION FACTS PER SERVING:
Total carbs: 9.1 g / Fiber: 3.2 g / Net carbs: 5.9 g / Protein: 37.9 g / Fat: 30.3 g / Calories: 463 kcal
Macronutrient ratio: Calories from carbs (5%), protein (34%), fat (61%)

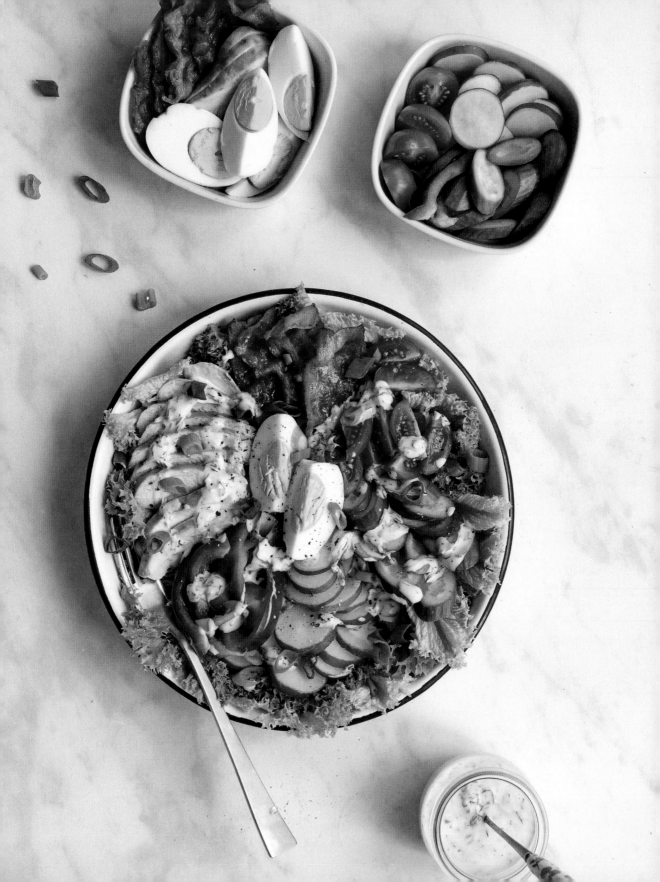

Chapter 6
Lunch Box

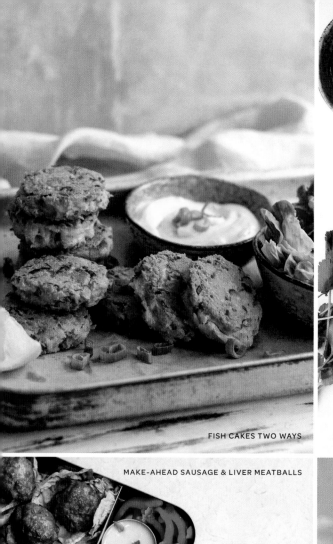

FISH CAKES TWO WAYS

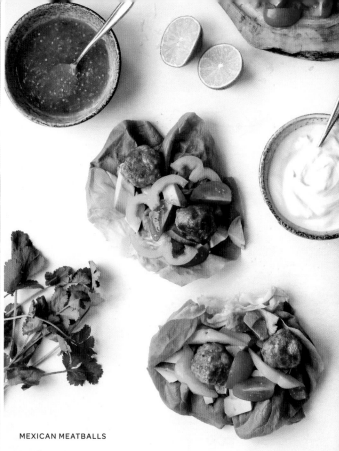

MEXICAN MEATBALLS

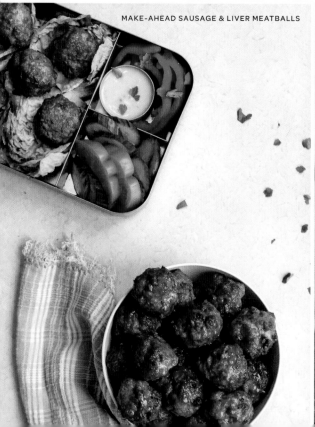

MAKE-AHEAD SAUSAGE & LIVER MEATBALLS

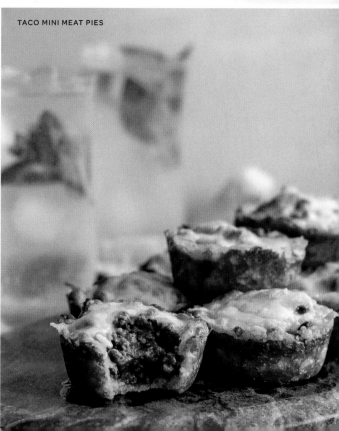

TACO MINI MEAT PIES

Bacon Caprese Egg Cups

SERVINGS: 6
HANDS-ON TIME: 10 minutes
OVERALL TIME: 30 minutes

These Caprese-style bacon egg cups are the perfect packable lunch. Grab one, two, or three cups and place them in your lunch box with chopped salads. Or simply serve them with dressed greens.

9 slices (290 g/10.2 oz) bacon
(about 32 g/1.1 oz each)

4 large eggs

½ cup (45 g/1.5 oz) grated Parmesan cheese

10 basil leaves, chopped

Pinch of salt and pepper

3½ ounces (100 g) fresh mozzarella, cut into 6 pieces

3 small (28 g/1 oz) cherry tomatoes, halved

Optional: 1 tablespoon (15 ml) extra-virgin olive oil and more basil

Preheat the oven to 430°F (220°C) forced fan or 465°F (240°C) conventional.

Place 1½ slices of bacon in the holes of a medium-size muffin pan to create 6 cups. Place in the oven and bake for about 12 minutes. Remove from the oven and drain any excess fat and juices. You can use a piece of paper towel to soak up any juices.

While the bacon is in the oven, crack the eggs into a bowl. Add the Parmesan cheese, basil, salt, and pepper, and whisk until well combined. Divide the egg mixture evenly among the 6 cups. Top each one with a piece of fresh mozzarella and half a cherry tomato.

Place back in the oven and bake for another 10 to 12 minutes. Optionally, drizzle with olive oil and sprinkle with more basil. Eat warm or cold. To store, keep in a sealed jar in the fridge for up to 4 days or freeze for up to 3 months.

NUTRITION FACTS PER SERVING (1 BACON CUP):
Total carbs: 1.1 g / Fiber: 0.1 g / Net carbs: 1 g / Protein: 17.6 g / Fat: 19.9 g / Calories: 256 kcal
Macronutrient ratio: Calories from carbs (2%), protein (28%), fat (70%)

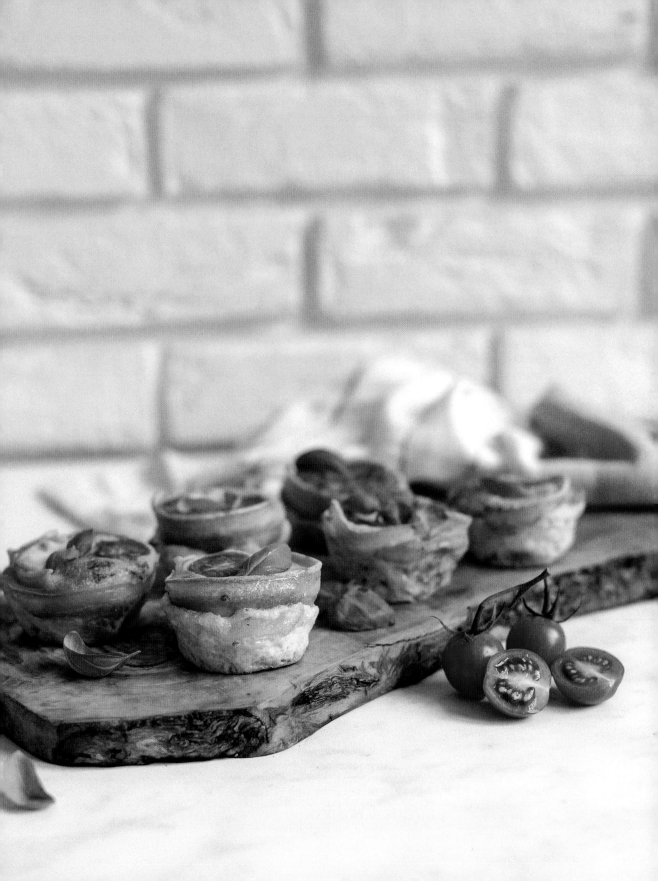

Unwich Two Ways

SERVINGS: 1
HANDS-ON TIME: 5 minutes
OVERALL TIME: 5 minutes

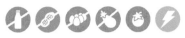

Unwich is the perfect grab-n-go meal. It takes just a few minutes to prepare, and it will fit perfectly in your lunch box!

4 soft green lettuce leaves (60 g/2.1 oz)

HAM & CHEESE UNWICH

1 tablespoon (15 g/0.5 oz) mayonnaise (page 16)
½ teaspoon lemon juice
1 tablespoon chopped herbs, such as parsley, dill, or chives
1 teaspoon tomato paste
4 slices (85 g/3 oz) quality ham
2 slices (57 g/2 oz) cheese such as provolone, Gouda, or Cheddar
4 radishes (60 g/2.1 oz), sliced

AVOCADO & EGG UNWICH

1½ tablespoons (23 g/0.8 oz) mayonnaise (page 16)
½ teaspoon lemon juice
1 tablespoon chopped herbs, such as parsley, dill, or chives (plus more for serving)
½ teaspoon Dijon or whole-grain mustard
2 large hard-boiled eggs, quartered (see page 15)
½ large (100 g/3.5 oz) avocado, sliced

Prepare the dressing by mixing the mayo, lemon juice, and chopped herbs for your choice of unwich. Add the tomato paste (for the ham & cheese version) or Dijon mustard (for the avocado & egg).

Place a piece of parchment or aluminum foil down. Place the lettuce on top in a single layer slightly overlapping.

TO MAKE THE HAM & CHEESE UNWICH: Add the ham, cheese, and radishes. Drizzle with the prepared dressing.

TO MAKE THE AVOCADO & EGG UNWICH: Add the egg and avocado. Drizzle with the prepared dressing and add chopped herbs to taste.

TO ASSEMBLE THE UNWICH: Roll the wrap tightly, tucking the edges like a sushi roll, pulling the parchment up and out as you fold it over so you're not tucking the paper into the wrap. Once wrapped, cut in half with a sharp knife. To eat, simply pull the parchment away as you go. Store in the fridge for up to 1 day.

TIP:

Instead of radishes, use sliced bell peppers, tomatoes, or cucumber. Instead of mayonnaise, use full-fat sour cream.

NUTRITION FACTS PER SERVING (HAM & CHEESE/AVOCADO & EGG):
Total carbs: 6.2/11.7 g / Fiber: 1.9/7.8 g / Net carbs: 4.3/3.9 g / Protein: 30.3/15.8 g / Fat: 30.4/43.1 g / Calories: 415/482 kcal
Macronutrient ratio: Calories from carbs (4/3%), protein (29/14%), fat (67/83%)

Nori Wraps Two Ways

SERVINGS: 1
HANDS-ON TIME: 5 minutes
OVERALL TIME: 5 minutes

I love using nori sheets as wraps because they are packed with flavor and are virtually zero carb. They work with pretty much any filling that is not too moist, as the nori gets soggy and may fall apart.

1 nori sheet

1 large or 2 small (20 g/1.4 oz) chard leaves or soft lettuce, thick stems cut off

SALMON NORI WRAPS

1½ tablespoons (23 g/0.8 oz) mayonnaise (page 16)

1 teaspoon fresh lemon juice

4 ounces (115 g) drained canned salmon

Salt and pepper, to taste

½ medium (75 g/2.7 oz) avocado, sliced

SARDINE NORI WRAPS

1½ tablespoons (23 g/0.8 oz) mayonnaise (page 16)

½ teaspoon Dijon or whole-grain mustard

4 ounces (115 g) drained canned sardines

¼ small (15 g/0.5 oz) red onion, diced

Salt and pepper, to taste

½ small (45 g/1.5 oz) cucumber, cut into matchsticks

To assemble, place the nori sheet on a chopping board. Add the chard leaves.

TO MAKE THE SALMON NORI WRAPS: In a small bowl, mix the mayo with the lemon juice. Add the salmon and combine well. Season to taste. Place on top of the chard leaves and add the avocado slices.

TO MAKE THE SARDINE NORI WRAPS: In a small bowl, mix the mayo with the mustard. Add the sardines and the onion and combine well. Season to taste. Place on top of the chard leaves and add the cucumber sticks.

Make sure you leave some space on each side of the nori sheet. Fold the long sides of the nori over the filling. Roll the wrap tight and wet the edges of the nori to help it hold together. Secure with a toothpick, if necessary. These are best eaten fresh but can be stored in the fridge for up to 2 days.

TIPS:

• Swap the filling for ham & cheese (page 94), avocado & egg (page 94), buffalo chicken (page 96), or shrimp & chorizo (page 96). Or try mackerel or spicy tuna (simply use canned fish and add 1 teaspoon of sriracha sauce).

• Are you egg-free? Swap the mayo for crème fraîche or sour cream.

NUTRITION FACTS PER SERVING (SALMON/SARDINE NORI WRAPS):
Total carbs: 11.4/5.8 g / Fiber: 8.2/2.4 g / Net carbs: 3.2/3.4 g / Protein: 34.2/31 g / Fat: 40.3/32.3 g / Calories: 521/436 kcal
Macronutrient ratio: Calories from carbs (3/3%), protein (27/29%), fat (70/68%)

Chard Wraps Two Ways

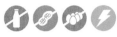

SERVINGS: 2
HANDS-ON TIME: 10 minutes
OVERALL TIME: 10 minutes

These wraps are so easy to put together. You can use any protein, dressing, and veggies for the filling. They are similar to Unwiches (page 94) but I used chard instead of lettuce. Feel free to use soft lettuce instead!

6 chard leaves (120 g/4.2 oz) with stems removed, or soft lettuce leaves

BUFFALO CHICKEN WRAPS
2 tablespoons (30 ml) buffalo sauce or sriracha
2 tablespoons (30 ml) melted butter
1 teaspoon coconut aminos or tamari
1 teaspoon white wine vinegar or apple cider vinegar
¼ teaspoon garlic powder
2 small (170 g/6 oz) cooked chicken breasts, shredded
2 medium (30 g/1.1 oz) spring onions, sliced
½ cup (68 g/2.4 oz) crumbled blue cheese

SHRIMP & CHORIZO WRAPS
½ cup (57 g/2 oz) diced Spanish chorizo or pepperoni
½ small (35 g/1.2 oz) yellow onion, sliced
5 ounces (140 g) cooked shrimp, chopped
1 teaspoon fresh lime or lemon juice
2 tablespoons (30 g/1.1 oz) mayonnaise (page 16)
¼ teaspoon chipotle chile powder or smoked paprika
½ large (100 g/5.3 oz) avocado, sliced or diced
1 tablespoon (4 g/0.2 oz) chopped cilantro or parsley

FOR THE BUFFALO CHICKEN WRAPS: Prepare the dressing by mixing the buffalo sauce, melted butter, coconut aminos, vinegar, and garlic powder in a bowl. Add the shredded chicken and mix to combine so that the chicken is well coated. Mix in the spring onions and crumbled blue cheese.

FOR THE SHRIMP & CHORIZO WRAPS: Heat a medium skillet over medium-high heat and add the chorizo. Cook for about 1 minute, until fragrant and the juices start to release. Add the onion and cook for 5 minutes. Take off the heat, place the filling in a mixing bowl, and let it cool slightly. Add the cooked shrimp, lime juice, mayo, and chile powder. Mix to combine. Finally, add the avocado and herbs.

TO ASSEMBLE THE WRAPS: Place a piece of parchment or aluminum foil down. Place the chard on top in a single layer slightly overlapping. Add the filling. Roll the wrap tightly, tucking the edges like a sushi roll, pulling the parchment up and out as you fold it over so you're not tucking the paper into the wrap. Once wrapped, cut in half with a sharp knife. To eat, simply pull the parchment away as you go. (1 wrap = both halves per serving.)

NUTRITION FACTS PER SERVING (1 BUFFALO CHICKEN/SHRIMP & CHORIZO WRAP):
Total carbs: 6.3/9.7 g / Fiber: 1.7/5 g / Net carbs: 4.6/4.7 g / Protein: 33.8/23.6 g / Fat: 24.8/32.3 g / Calories: 383/417 kcal
Macronutrient ratio: Calories from carbs (5/5%), protein (36/23%), fat (59/72%)

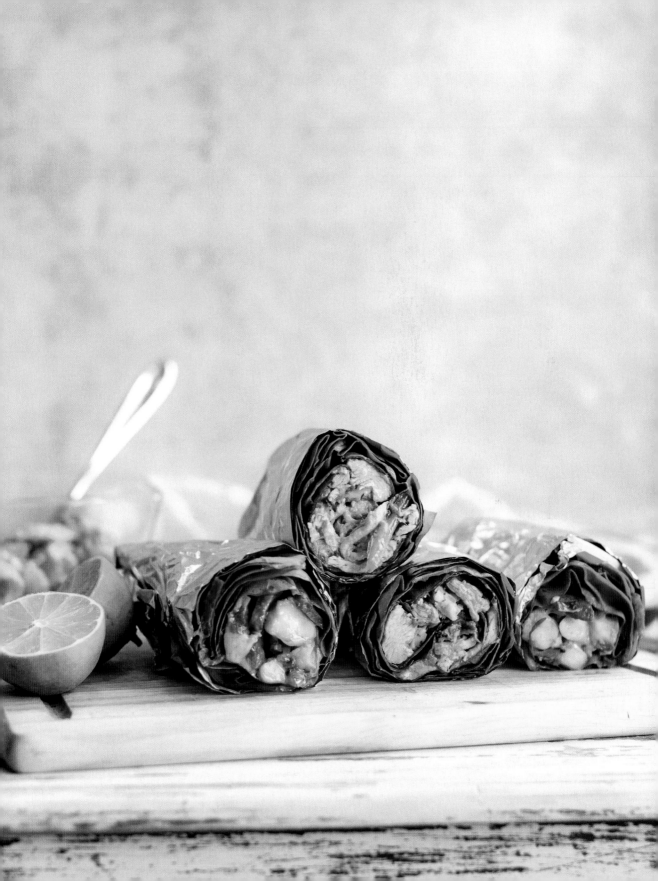

Cheesy Muffins Two Ways

SERVINGS: 10 muffins
HANDS-ON TIME: 10 minutes
OVERALL TIME: 30 to 40 minutes

This recipe was an accidental experiment. I was planning to make savory cheese muffins for a family gathering and added some leftover breakfast sausage. I thought it would be a fun snack to make and the kids loved it! It ended up being the kind of recipe my partner asks for over and over again, and I love making it because it's so easy. I included a veggie option with feta too!

SAUSAGE MUFFINS

7 ounces (200 g) gluten-free Italian-style sausages

¼ cup (60 ml) melted ghee or butter, plus extra for greasing

4 large eggs

Pinch of black pepper

1 teaspoon onion powder

¼ teaspoon garlic powder

1 cup (113 g/4 oz) shredded Cheddar cheese

½ cup (50 g/1.8 oz) almond flour

¼ cup (30 g/1.1 oz) coconut flour

1 teaspoon gluten-free baking powder

2 medium (30 g/1.1 oz) spring onions, sliced

FETA MUFFINS

4 large eggs

¼ cup (60 ml) melted ghee or butter

Pinch of black pepper

1 teaspoon onion powder

¼ teaspoon garlic powder

1 cup (90 g/3.2 oz) grated Parmesan cheese

½ cup (50 g/1.8 oz) almond flour

¼ cup (30 g/1.1 oz) coconut flour

1 teaspoon gluten-free baking powder

20 pitted black or green olives (60 g/2.1 oz), sliced

2 tablespoons (8 g/0.3 oz) fresh herbs, such as oregano, basil, and thyme (Or use 2 teaspoons [2 g] dried Italian herbs.)

7 ounces (200 g) feta cheese, cut into 10 pieces, or use soft goat's cheese

Preheat the oven to 350°F (175°C) forced fan or 380°F (195°C) conventional.

TO MAKE THE SAUSAGE MUFFINS: Place the sausages in a hot pan lightly greased with ghee and cook over medium heat for 5 to 10 minutes, until browned on all sides. When done, let them cool down and cut to make 10 pieces, one for each muffin.

TO MAKE BOTH MUFFINS: Crack the eggs into a bowl, add the melted ghee, and whisk until combined. Add all the remaining ingredients apart from the sausage (for sausage muffins) or feta (for feta muffins).

Scoop the dough into a medium-size muffin pan and fill 10 muffin holes. Each should be about three-quarters full. Finally, add a piece of sausage (for sausage muffins) or feta (for feta muffins) in the middle of each.

Place in the oven and bake for 20 to 25 minutes. The tops should be lightly browned and the dough set. Eat warm or cold. Store in the fridge for up to 5 days or freeze for up to 3 months.

TIP:

Are you nut-free? Swap the ½ cup (50 g/1.8 oz) almond flour for 2 tablespoons (16 g/0.6 oz) coconut flour or 4 tablespoons (28 g/1 oz) flax meal.

NUTRITION FACTS PER SERVING (1 SAUSAGE MUFFIN/FETA MUFFIN):
Total carbs: 2.8/3.6 g / Fiber: 1.1/1.3 g / Net carbs: 1.7/2.3 g / Protein: 7.1/7.8 g / Fat: 18.6/16 g / Calories: 208/190 kcal
Macronutrient ratio: Calories from carbs (3/5%), protein (14/17%), fat (83/78%)

Mini Cheeseburger Parcels

SERVINGS: 5 (10 parcels total)
HANDS-ON TIME: 10 minutes
OVERALL TIME: 20 minutes

These mini cheeseburger parcels taste like your favorite cheeseburger with none of the carbs. They are perfect for lunch boxes or as a cute party snack! Optionally, serve these with more mustard and ketchup, and with salad or roasted veggies.

1 pound (450 g) ground beef

1 tablespoon (15 g/0.5 oz) Dijon mustard

2 tablespoons (30 g/1.1 oz) tomato paste or sugar-free ketchup

1 tablespoon (7 g/0.3 oz) onion powder

½ teaspoon salt

¼ teaspoon black pepper

10 slices (150 g/5.3 oz) Parma ham

2½ small (60 g/2.1 oz) pickles, cut into quarters

2½ ounces (70 g) Cheddar cheese, cut into 10 pieces

Preheat the oven to 400°F (200°C) forced fan or 425°F (220°C) conventional. Line a baking dish with parchment paper or a silicone mat.

In a bowl, mix the beef, Dijon mustard, tomato paste, onion powder, salt, and pepper. Lay a slice of Parma ham on a cutting board. Place about 50 g (1.8 oz) of the meat mixture on the slice. Press a piece of pickle and Cheddar into the meat. Wrap the Parma ham slice around the meat and place it in the baking dish cheese-and-pickle side up. Repeat for all the remaining 9 pieces.

Bake for about 10 minutes. Eat warm (2 parcels per serving). Store in the fridge for up to 4 days and reheat before serving.

TIPS:

• Swap Parma ham for pancetta or bacon!

• If you can't find keto-approved ketchup, you can easily make your own. Check out my recipes at ketodietapp.com/blog for homemade condiments, including ketchup, BBQ sauce, mustard, chile paste, etc.

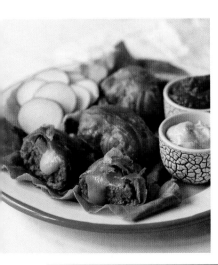

NUTRITION FACTS PER SERVING (2 PARCELS):
Total carbs: 2 g / Fiber: 0.6 g / Net carbs: 2.6 g / Protein: 26.8 g / Fat: 26.3 g / Calories: 361 kcal
Macronutrient ratio: Calories from carbs (2%), protein (30%), fat (68%)

Fish Cakes Two Ways

SERVINGS: 2 (6 patties total)
HANDS-ON TIME: 10 minutes
OVERALL TIME: 30 minutes

I can never get bored of fish cakes because there are a thousand ways to make them and they can be adjusted to almost any preference. They are the perfect packable snack that can be scaled up and made several days in advance. I like to serve them with leafy greens and high-fat dips.

2 tablespoons (30 ml) ghee, duck fat, or coconut oil for frying

THAI COD FISH CAKES

8.8 ounces (250 g) cod, skinless and boneless

2 tablespoons (30 g/1.1 oz) Thai curry paste, or to taste

1 large egg

¼ teaspoon salt

¼ teaspoon pepper

1 tablespoon (8 g/0.3 oz) coconut flour

2 medium (30 g/1.1 oz) spring onions, sliced

1 tablespoon (4 g/0.2 oz) chopped cilantro or parsley

TUNA FISH CAKES

8.8 ounces (250 g) drained canned tuna

2 teaspoons (10 ml) fresh lemon juice

1 large egg

¼ small (15 g/0.5 oz) red onion, finely chopped

¼ teaspoon salt

¼ teaspoon black pepper

3 tablespoons (15 g/0.5 oz) grated Parmesan cheese

¼ cup (25 g/0.9 oz) almond flour

1 medium (15 g/0.5 oz) spring onion, sliced, or chopped chives

TO MAKE THE THAI COD FISH CAKES: Place all the ingredients except the ghee, spring onion, and parsley in a blender. Process until smooth. Add the spring onion and cilantro and stir through.

TO MAKE THE TUNA CAKES: Place all the ingredients except the ghee in a mixing bowl and combine.

TO COOK THE FISH CAKES: Use a ¼-cup measuring cup (about 60 g/2.1 oz) to measure out each patty. The mixture will be wet, so you'll need to use your hands to form the patties.

Heat a large pan greased with the ghee over medium heat. Once hot, add as many patties as you can fit in a single layer, until you've cooked 6 patties in total. Cook them on each side for about 5 minutes and use a spatula to flip them over. Do not force the patties out of the pan: if a patty doesn't release when you try to flip it, cook it for a few more seconds until it's crisp and ready to flip. Set the cooked patties aside.

Serve with high-fat dips such as aioli or ranch dressing (page 88). Store in the fridge in a sealed contained for up to 4 days or freeze for up to 3 months.

TIPS:

• Are you egg-free or nut-free? Swap the egg for chia egg (page 15). They are not the perfect substitute for eggs, but you'll get decent results. For nut-free, you can swap the ¼ cup (25 g/0.9 oz) almond flour for 1 tablespoon (8 g/0.3 oz) coconut flour.

• For homemade Thai curry paste, check out my recipes at ketodietapp.com/blog.

PICTURED ON PAGE 91

NUTRITION FACTS PER SERVING (3 THAI FISH CAKES/TUNA FISH CAKES):
Total carbs: 6.4/4.4 g / Fiber: 2.4/1.7 g / Net carbs: 4/2.7 g / Protein: 27.6/33.1 g / Fat: 19.6/27.1 g / Calories: 322/389 kcal
Macronutrient ratio: Calories from carbs (5/3%), protein (36/34%), fat (59/63%)

Taco Mini Meat Pies

SERVINGS: 10 mini pies
HANDS-ON TIME: 15 minutes
OVERALL TIME: 30 minutes

This is one of my absolute favorite recipes from this book. The taco sauce takes no more than 15 minutes to make—and then you are only four ingredients away from amazing keto meat pies!

14.1 ounces (400 g) ground beef

⅓ cup (80 ml) sugar-free taco sauce (see tip)

1½ cups (170 g/6 oz) low-moisture shredded mozzarella

⅔ cup (66 g/2.3 oz) almond flour

1 cup (113 g/4 oz) grated Cheddar or more mozzarella

Optional: sugar-free ketchup or mustard

Heat a large skillet over medium-high heat. Add the beef and taco sauce, and cook for 5 to 8 minutes, until browned on all sides. Melt the mozzarella in the microwave for 1 minute or in a saucepan over low heat. Mix and add the almond flour. Stir until the dough is well combined.

Preheat the oven to 350°F (175°C) forced fan or 380°F (195°C) conventional.

Cut the dough into 4 equal pieces. Use an 8-hole medium-size muffin pan and press the dough into each cup. Be sure to leave overhang at the top; the dough will shrink while cooking. Bake for about 10 minutes.

Remove from the oven and use a spoon to flatten the slightly inflated cups. Add the beef filling, and top with the Cheddar cheese. Return to the oven and bake for another 8 to 10 minutes. Eat warm, optionally with sugar-free ketchup or mustard. Store in the fridge for up to 4 days or freeze for up to 3 months.

TIPS:

• Are you nut-free? Swap the ⅔ cup (66 g/2.3 oz) almond flour for ½ cup (75 g) packed flax meal, or 6 tablespoons (24 g/0.8 oz) coconut flour. If you use any of the nut-free alternatives, you will need to add ¼ cup (57 g/2 oz) cream cheese to the mozzarella before microwaving.

• To make the DIY Taco Sauce (about 1¾ cups/415 ml): Place the following ingredients in a saucepan: 1 cup (240 ml) tomato sauce, 2 tablespoons (30 ml) apple cider vinegar, 1 tablespoon (5 g/0.2 oz) ground cumin, ½ cup (120 ml) water, 1 teaspoon onion powder, ½ teaspoon garlic powder, 1 teaspoon dried oregano, 1 teaspoon Mexican chile powder of choice, 1 teaspoon sweet or smoked paprika, 2 to 3 teaspoons erythritol or Swerve (or 3 to 6 drops of stevia), ¼ teaspoon cayenne pepper, 1 teaspoon salt or to taste. Bring to a boil and cook over medium-low heat for 7 to 10 minutes, until reduced and thickened slightly. Store in the fridge in a sealed jar for up to a week or freeze in an ice cube tray for up to 6 months.

PICTURED ON PAGE 91

NUTRITION FACTS PER SERVING (1 MINI MEAT PIE):
Total carbs: 3 g / Fiber: 0.8 g / Net carbs: 2.2 g / Protein: 15 g / Fat: 18.7 g / Calories: 239 kcal
Macronutrient ratio: Calories from carbs (4%), protein (25%), fat (71%)

Turkey Parmesan Patties

SERVINGS: 5 (20 small patties total)
HANDS-ON TIME: 20 minutes
OVERALL TIME: 20 minutes

This healthy low-carb meal is quick to prepare and perfect for batch cooking. Simply make the patties on a Sunday and you've got a healthy lunch option ready for the whole week! Serve them with some aioli or ranch dressing (page 88) and roasted veggies or fresh salad. Or try them with Italian Cauli-Rice (page 63). They are freezer-friendly, so you can scale up and make a large batch, too.

1.1 pounds (500 g) ground turkey or chicken

1 cup (90 g/3.2 oz) grated Parmesan cheese

1 large egg

1 clove garlic, crushed

2 tablespoons (8 g/0.3 oz) fresh herbs (basil, dill, chives, thyme, or parsley) or 2 teaspoons (2 g/0.1 oz) dried Italian herbs

½ teaspoon salt

¼ teaspoon black pepper

2 tablespoons (30 ml) ghee or duck fat

Place all the ingredients for the patties, except for the ghee, in a bowl. Mix until well combined. Make 20 small patties (about 32 g/1.1 oz each) or 15 medium-size patties (about 43 g/1.5 oz each).

Heat a large skillet greased with ghee over medium-high heat. Once hot, add as many patties as you can fit in a single layer. Cook them on each side for 4 to 5 minutes and use a spatula to flip them over. Do not force the patties out of the pan: if a patty doesn't release when you try to flip it, cook it for a few more seconds until it's crisp and ready to flip. Set the cooked patties aside, and repeat until you've cooked all the patties. Serve with high-fat dips such as aioli or ranch dressing (page 88). Store in the fridge in a sealed contained for up to 4 days or freeze for up to 3 months.

TIPS:

• Instead of frying the patties, you can bake them in the oven in a muffin pan by placing each patty into each muffin hole greased with ghee. Bake at 400°F (200°C) forced fan or 425°F (220°C) conventional for about 15 minutes, or until lightly golden.

• Are you egg-free? Swap the egg for chia egg (page 15). They are not the perfect substitute for eggs, but you'll get decent results.

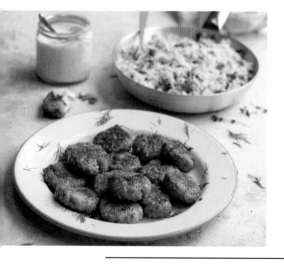

NUTRITION FACTS PER SERVING (4 SMALL/3 MEDIUM PATTIES):
Total carbs: 1.2 g / Fiber: 0.2 g / Net carbs: 1 g / Protein: 24.7 g / Fat: 24.2 g / Calories: 322 kcal
Macronutrient ratio: Calories from carbs (1%), protein (31%), fat (68%)

Mexican Meatballs

SERVINGS: 5 (25 meatballs total)
HANDS-ON TIME: 20 minutes
OVERALL TIME: 20 minutes

Life can get really busy. When it does, keeping your meals simple is key to a successful low-carb diet. And it's no different for me. Even as a food blogger, I don't always have the time to cook. But instead of reaching for quick snacks, I have a routine that helps me stay keto. When I'm short on time, I prep my protein in advance. Making a large freezer-friendly batch of meatballs is one great way to do it!

MEATBALLS

1.1 pounds (500 g) ground pork, 15% fat

5 ounces (140 g) Mexican chorizo

1 large egg

¾ cup (75 g/2.7 oz) almond flour

1 teaspoon dried oregano

½ teaspoon salt

¼ teaspoon black pepper

1 tablespoon (15 ml) ghee, duck fat, or lard

TO SERVE

Sliced avocado, tomatoes, peppers, and cucumbers

Serve as tacos on lettuce leaves

Sour cream or full-fat yogurt

Salsa Verde (see tip) or guacamole

Fresh cilantro and lime wedges

TO MAKE THE MEATBALLS: In a bowl, mix all the ingredients for the meatballs except for the ghee. Using your hands, create 25 small meatballs (about 31 g/1.1 oz each).

Heat a large skillet greased with ghee over high heat. Once hot, reduce the heat to medium-high and add the meatballs. Cook for about 2 minutes, or until crisp, and turn onto the other side using a fork. Cook for another 2 minutes, or until cooked through.

Serve warm with the accompaniments of your choice or let them cool down and refrigerate for up to 4 days or freeze for up to 3 months.

TIPS:

- To make Salsa Verde (makes about 1½ cups/360 ml): Place the following ingredients in a blender: 1 cup (28 g/1 oz) packed fresh basil, 2 cups (50 g/1.8 oz) fresh parsley, ¼ cup (6 g/0.2 oz) fresh mint, 2 tablespoons (17 g/0.6 oz) drained capers, 4 canned anchovy fillets (16 g/0.6 oz), 2 cloves garlic (sliced), 3 tablespoons (45 ml) apple cider vinegar, 2 tablespoons (30 ml) fresh lemon juice, ¾ cup (180 ml) extra-virgin olive oil, 1 teaspoon salt, and ½ teaspoon black pepper (or to taste). Process until smooth or chunky. Store in a sealed jar in the fridge for up to 2 weeks.

- Are you egg-free? Swap the egg for chia egg (page 15). They are not the perfect substitute for eggs, but you'll get decent results.

- Are you nut-free? Swap the ¾ cup (85 g/3 oz) almond flour for ¼ cup (30 g/1.1 oz) coconut flour.

PICTURED ON PAGE 91

NUTRITION FACTS PER SERVING (5 MEATBALLS):
Total carbs: 4.5 g / Fiber: 2 g / Net carbs: 2.5 g / Protein: 27 g / Fat: 33.4 g / Calories: 421 kcal
Macronutrient ratio: Calories from carbs (2%), protein (26%), fat (72%)

Make-Ahead Sausage & Liver Meatballs

SERVINGS: 5 (25 meatballs total)
HANDS-ON TIME: 20 minutes
OVERALL TIME: 20 minutes

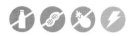

There are so many reasons why I love liver. It's a superfood that is rich in vitamin A, vitamin B$_{12}$, and copper, plus high-quality protein. Even if you're not a fan of organ meats, these meatballs are a great way to start because chicken livers have a mild flavor and are masked with sausage and Parmesan in this recipe. I used homemade sausage meat because it's easy to make. You can always use store-bought sausage meat instead of homemade—just watch out for added starches and sugar.

HOMEMADE SAUSAGE MEAT

1.7 pounds (750 g) ground pork, 15% fat

3 cloves garlic, crushed

¾ teaspoon dried sage

¾ teaspoon thyme

½ teaspoon dried fennel seeds

⅛ teaspoon ground nutmeg

⅛ teaspoon ground cloves

¾ teaspoon salt

½ teaspoon black pepper

SAUSAGE & LIVER MEATBALLS

½ batch (385 g/13.6 oz) Homemade Sausage Meat (recipe above)

6 ounces (170 g) chicken livers, finely chopped

1 cup (90 g/3.2 oz) grated Parmesan cheese

1 large egg

½ teaspoon salt

2 tablespoons (30 ml) ghee, duck fat, or lard for frying

TO MAKE THE SAUSAGE MEAT: In a bowl, mix all the ingredients for the sausage meat. Place half of the sausage meat (385 g/13.6 oz) in a plastic bag and freeze for later, up to 3 months.

TO MAKE THE MEATBALLS: Mix the remaining sausage meat with the chicken livers, cheese, egg, and salt. Using your hands, create 25 small meatballs (about 28 g/1 oz each).

Heat a large skillet greased with ghee over high heat. Once hot, reduce the heat to medium-high and add the meatballs. Cook for about 2 minutes, or until crisp. Turn on the other side using a fork and cook for another 2 minutes, or until cooked through.

Serve warm or let them cool down and refrigerate for up to 4 days.

TIPS:

- Did you know that apart from plant foods, chicken liver is a great source of vitamin C? If your carb intake is very low, consider adding chicken liver to your diet.
- If you're new to organ meats, use mild-tasting chicken or turkey livers. Instead of chicken liver you can use calf liver, beef, pork, or lamb liver.

PICTURED ON PAGE 91

NUTRITION FACTS PER SERVING (5 MEATBALLS):
Total carbs: 1.8 g / Fiber: 0.2 g / Net carbs: 1.6 g / Protein: 27 g / Fat: 25.3 g / Calories: 346 kcal
Macronutrient ratio: Calories from carbs (2%), protein (32%), fat (66%)

Shrimp Fajita Lunch Bowls

SERVINGS: 2
HANDS-ON TIME: 15 minutes
OVERALL TIME: 15 minutes + marinating

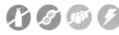

These tortilla-free fajitas are served "naked," just like bunless burgers! You can keep them simple or add your favorite Mexican toppings.

2 teaspoons fajita seasoning (see tip)

1 clove garlic, minced

¼ cup (60 ml) extra-virgin olive oil

2 tablespoons (30 ml) fresh lime juice

8.8 ounces (250 g) raw shrimp

½ medium (55 g/1.9 oz) yellow onion, sliced

1 small (75 g/2.5 oz) green bell pepper, sliced

1 medium (120 g/4.2 oz) red, yellow, or orange bell pepper, sliced

2 tablespoons (30 ml) ghee or more olive oil, divided

Fresh cilantro, to taste

Optional: cauli-rice (page 14), sliced avocado, sour cream, salsa (page 106), and lime wedges

TO MAKE THE MARINADE: Mix the fajita seasoning, garlic, olive oil, and lime juice in a bowl. Pour half (about 3 tablespoons/45 ml) of the marinade over the shrimp in a bowl and refrigerate for at least 1 hour or up to 24 hours. Pour the remaining marinade over the veggies. (You can also use two resealable plastic bags for this step.)

When ready to cook, drain the marinade from the shrimp. Grease a pan with 1 tablespoon (15 ml) of ghee, add the shrimp, and cook over high heat for 1 to 2 minutes, until the shrimp are opaque and lightly crisp—do not overcook. Remove from the pan and keep warm. Pour any leftover juices out of the pan and discard (part of the discarded marinade is not included in the nutrition facts).

Grease the same pan with the remaining 1 tablespoon (15 g) ghee and place over high heat. Add the vegetables, including the marinade, and cook for 3 to 5 minutes, stirring occasionally.

Serve the shrimp with the cooked vegetables and garnish with cilantro. Optionally serve with cauli-rice (page 14), avocado, sour cream, salsa, and lime wedges.

TIPS:

• You can make your own fajita seasoning. Simply mix ½ teaspoon Mexican chile powder, ½ teaspoon ground cumin, ¼ teaspoon red pepper flakes, ½ teaspoon salt, and ¼ teaspoon black pepper. That's it!

• For keto-approved homemade tortillas, visit ketodietapp.com/blog.

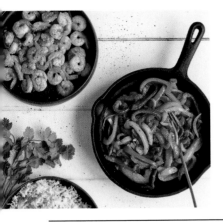

NUTRITION FACTS PER SERVING:
Total carbs: 11 g / Fiber: 3.1 g / Net carbs: 7.9 g / Protein: 19.7 g / Fat: 36.9 g / Calories: 446 kcal
Macronutrient ratio: Calories from carbs (7%), protein (18%), fat (75%)

Ground Beef Taco Bowl

SERVINGS: 4
HANDS-ON TIME: 20 minutes
OVERALL TIME: 20 minutes

Prep your protein and salsa in advance to save a ton of time. Then you'll only need a few minutes to reheat the meat and assemble the bowls!

SIMPLE SALSA

1–2 large (227 g/8 oz) tomatoes, ideally beefsteak tomatoes

½ small (35 g/1.2 oz) white onion, finely chopped

1 clove garlic, mined

1 jalapeño or serrano pepper (14 g/0.5 oz), seeds and ribs removed, minced

1 tablespoon (15 ml) fresh lime juice

1 tablespoon (4 g/0.2 oz) chopped cilantro or parsley

Salt and pepper, to taste

TACO BEEF

1 tablespoon (15 ml) ghee, duck fat, or olive oil

1.1 pounds (500 g) ground beef

⅔ cup (160 ml) Taco Sauce (page 101)

Salt and pepper, to taste

VEGGIES (PER SERVING)

4–6 leaves (85 g/3 oz) green lettuce

½ medium (75 g/2.7 oz) avocado, sliced

Cilantro

Lime wedges

Optional: a dollop of sour cream

TO MAKE THE SALSA: Finely dice the tomatoes and place in a mixing bowl. Beefsteak tomatoes are best because they contain fewer seeds. Add the onion, garlic, jalapeño pepper, lime juice, and cilantro. Mix and season with salt and pepper.

TO COOK THE BEEF: Heat a large skillet greased with ghee over medium-high heat. Add the beef and cook for about 5 minutes, until opaque. Add the taco sauce and cook for another 5 minutes, or until the juices are reduced. Season with salt and pepper.

TO ASSEMBLE THE BOWLS: Add the lettuce leaves to four bowls. Top with one-quarter of the cooked beef and one-quarter of the prepared salsa. Add avocado and serve with cilantro and lime wedges. The taco-flavored ground beef and salsa can be made up to 4 days in advance and stored in the fridge. Add a dollop of sour cream, if desired.

TIP:

You can easily create your own ground meat lunch bowls. For an Italian-style bowl, swap the taco sauce for Salsa Verde (page 103) or Simple Pesto (page 16). You can also try with Thai curry paste, chipotle chile paste, or harissa paste. Use any low-carb veggies, such as peppers, cucumber, radishes, or spinach, and swap the ground beef for ground chicken, turkey, pork, or lamb. The options are endless!

NUTRITION FACTS PER SERVING:
Total carbs: 14.4 g / Fiber: 7.7 g / Net carbs: 6.7 g / Protein: 25.2 g / Fat: 40.4 g / Calories: 514 kcal
Macronutrient ratio: Calories from carbs (5%), protein (21%), fat (74%)

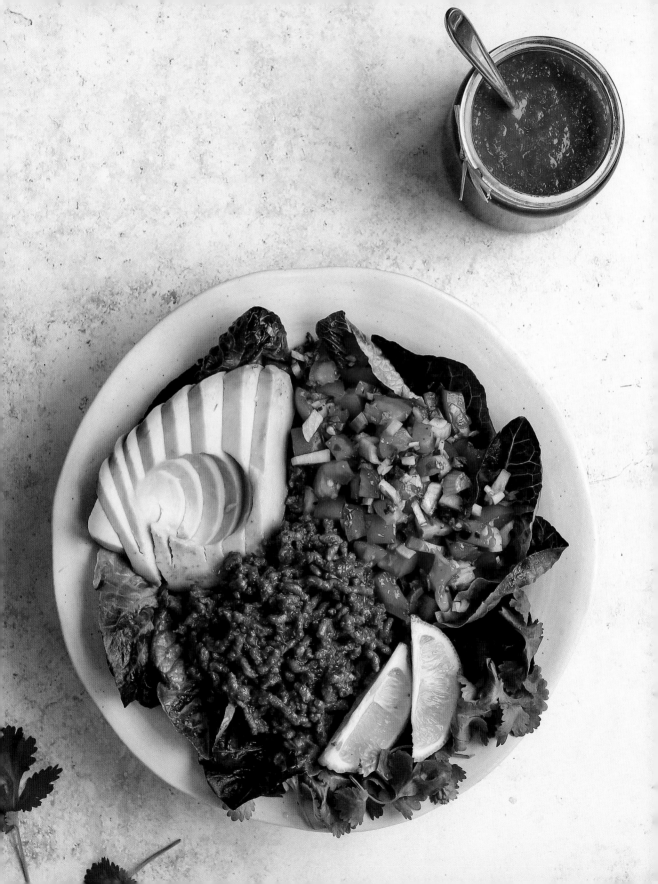

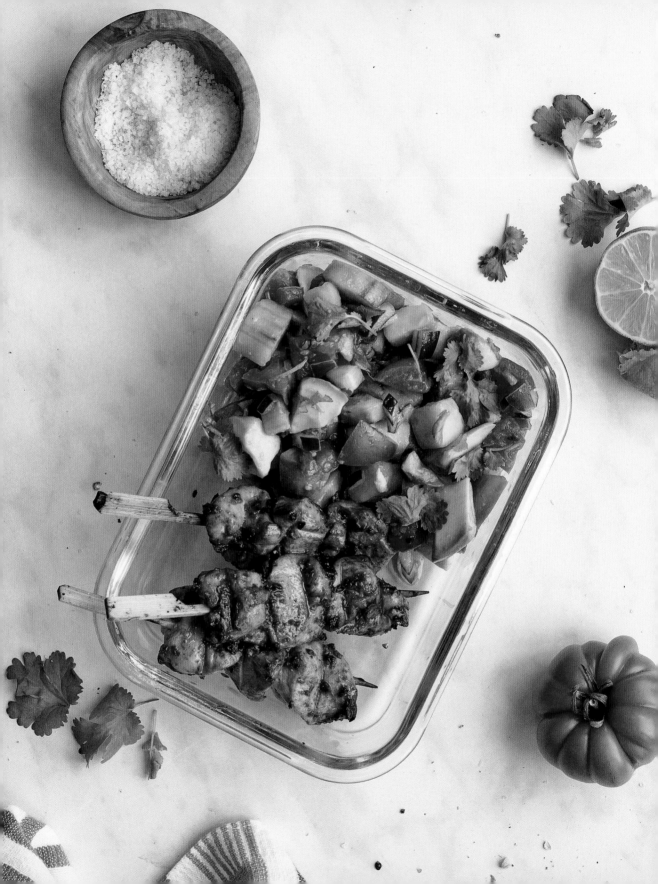

Chipotle Chicken Skewers with Chopped Salad

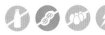

SERVINGS: 4 (8 skewers total)
HANDS-ON TIME: 20 minutes
OVERALL TIME: 20 minutes + marinating

Marinating chicken makes the meat juicy, tender, and full of flavor. It's simple and ideal for busy weeknights and healthy lunch boxes. Here it's served with a simple chopped salad. I used homemade Mexican chile paste. If you use store-bought, be sure to watch out for added sugar!

MARINATED CHICKEN

1.3 pounds (600 g) chicken breasts, cut into 1½-inch (4 cm) chunks
3 tablespoons (45 g/1.6 oz) chipotle chile paste or minced chipotle peppers in adobo (see tip)
¼ cup (60 ml) extra-virgin olive oil
1 tablespoon (15 ml) fresh lime juice
¼–½ teaspoon salt

EASY CHOPPED SALAD

¼ cup (60 ml) extra-virgin olive oil
1 tablespoon (15 ml) fresh lime juice
1 large (250 g/8.8 oz) cucumber, diced
1 large (200 g/7.1 oz) avocado, diced
½ medium (50 g/1.8 oz) red onion, diced
2 large (250 g/8.8 oz) tomatoes, diced
¼ cup (15 g/0.5 oz) chopped cilantro or parsley
Salt and pepper, to taste

TO MARINATE THE CHICKEN: Place the chicken chunks in a bowl. Add the chile paste, olive oil, lime juice, and salt. Mix until combined and marinate in the fridge for at least 1 hour or up to 24 hours. When you're ready to cook, line a baking sheet with aluminum foil and place a rack on top. Thread metal or soaked wooden skewers with the chicken chunks, 4 per skewer.

Preheat the oven to 430°F (220°C) forced fan or 465°F (240°C) conventional. Bake for 12 to 15 minutes, turning them halfway through and brushing with any leftover marinade from the bowl. When done, place on a cooling rack.

MEANWHILE, PREPARE THE SALSA: In a small bowl, whisk the olive oil and lime juice. Place the veggies in a mixing bowl. Pour the dressing over and mix to combine.

Serve with the skewers (about 1 cup/200 g/7.1 oz of salad with 2 skewers per serving).

TIP:

You can buy ready-made chipotle chile paste or use our keto-approved recipe. Find out more at ketodietapp.com/blog.

NUTRITION FACTS PER SERVING (ABOUT 1 CUP SALAD + 2 SKEWERS):
Total carbs: 13.2 g / Fiber: 4.9 g / Net carbs: 8.3 g / Protein: 34.6 g / Fat: 40.8 g / Calories: 560 kcal
Macronutrient ratio: Calories from carbs (6%), protein (27%), fat (67%)

Chapter 7

Dinners

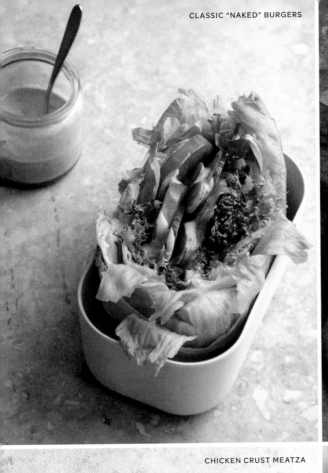
CLASSIC "NAKED" BURGERS

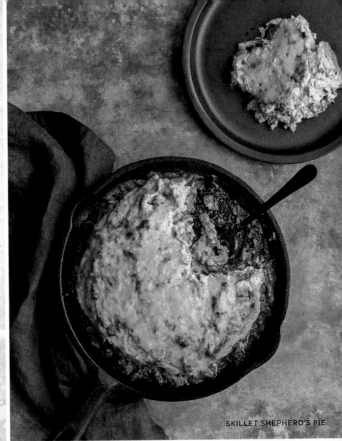
SKILLET SHEPHERD'S PIE

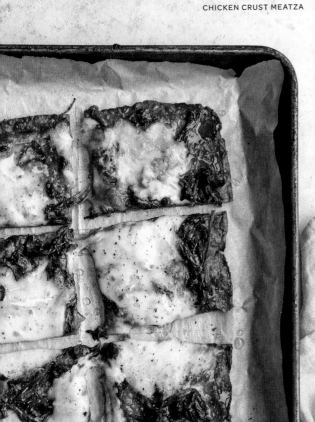
CHICKEN CRUST MEATZA

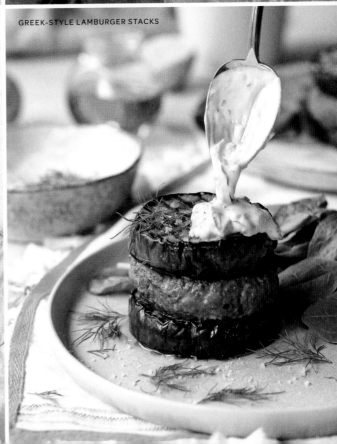
GREEK-STYLE LAMBURGER STACKS

Chicken Satay & Slaw Tray Bake

SERVINGS: 4
HANDS-ON TIME: 10 minutes
OVERALL TIME: 35 minutes

This chicken satay sheet pan is juicy, tender, and bursting with flavor. For maximum flavor I baked it like hasselback chicken—with slits filled with all that delicious satay sauce!

SAUCE

- 5 tablespoons (80 g / 2.8 oz) almond butter or peanut butter
- ⅓ cup (80 ml) extra-virgin olive oil or melted coconut oil
- 2 tablespoons (30 ml) coconut aminos or tamari
- 2 tablespoons (30 ml) fresh lime or lemon juice
- 1 tablespoon (15 ml) fish sauce or more coconut aminos
- 2 cloves garlic, minced
- ½ teaspoon red pepper flakes or 1 small (5 g / 0.2 oz) red chile pepper, minced
- 1 tablespoon (6 g / 0.2 oz) grated ginger or ¼– ½ teaspoon ground ginger

TRAY BAKE

- 4 medium (600 g / 1.3 lb.) chicken breasts, skinless and boneless (150 g / 5.3 oz each)
- Generous pinch of salt and pepper
- 1.1 pounds (500 g) coleslaw mix (you can use store-bought or make your own [page 71])
- 2 medium (30 g / 1.1 oz) spring onions, sliced
- Optional: fresh cilantro, peanuts, slivered almonds, or sesame seeds to sprinkle

TO MAKE THE SAUCE: Combine all the ingredients in a bowl. Set aside.

TO MAKE THE TRAY BAKE: Cut 5 to 7 slits widthwise into each breast, about ½ inch (1 cm) apart. Do not slice all the way through the breasts. Season each piece with salt and pepper. Place the chicken breasts on a baking tray. Using a spoon, pour about half of the sauce over the breasts and inside the slits. You can optionally marinate the chicken in the fridge for up to 24 hours.

Preheat the oven to 400°F (200°C) forced fan, or 425°F (220°C) conventional. Bake for about 15 minutes, and then remove from the oven. Push the breasts to one side and add the slaw. Drizzle with the remaining sauce and toss to combine. Place the chicken breasts on top of the slaw and bake for another 10 to 15 minutes. Serve warm, sprinkled with spring onions and any optional toppings. To store, refrigerate for up to 4 days.

TIP:

Are you nut-free? Swap the almond butter for sunflower seed butter or coconut butter (aka coconut manna, not to be confused with coconut cream or coconut oil).

NUTRITION FACTS PER SERVING:
Total carbs: 14 g / Fiber: 5.4 g / Net carbs: 8.6 g / Protein: 40 g / Fat: 33.2 g / Calories: 505 kcal
Macronutrient ratio: Calories from carbs (7%), protein (32%), fat (61%)

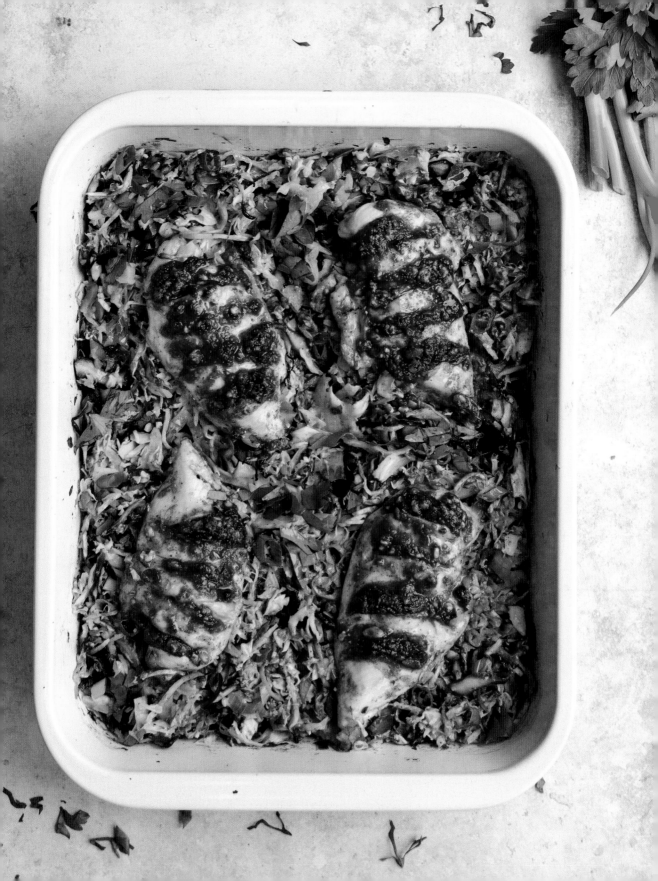

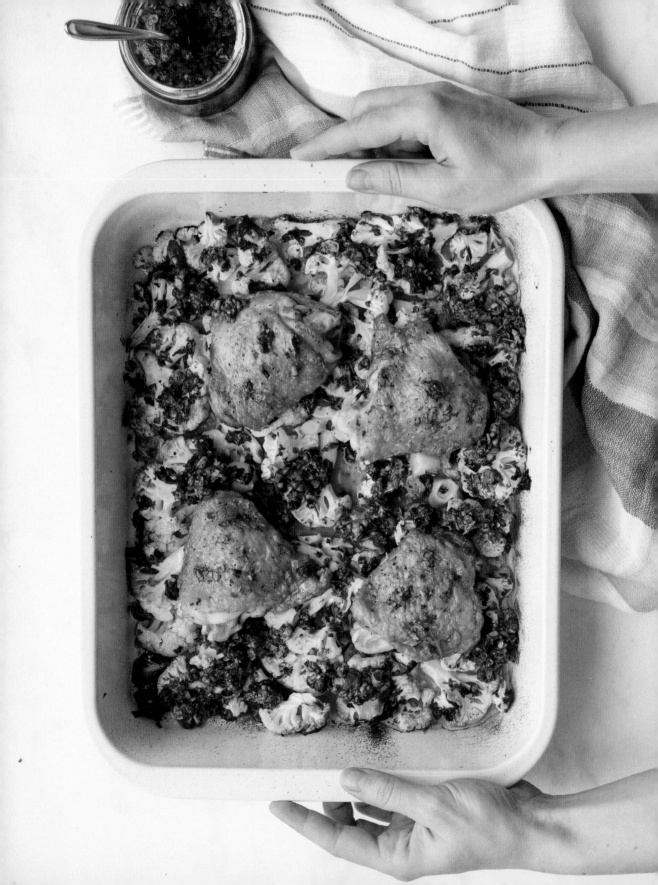

Salsa Verde Chicken Tray Bake

SERVINGS: 4
HANDS-ON TIME: 15 minutes
OVERALL TIME: 40 minutes

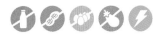

A simple Italian-inspired keto sheet pan made with easy five-minute salsa verde, crispy chicken thighs, and roasted cauliflower. This is perfect as a weekday treat!

1 medium (600 g/ 1.3 lb.) cauliflower

1 cup (240 ml) Salsa Verde (page 103), divided

4 large or 8 small (900 g/ 2 lb.) bone-in chicken thighs

Pinch of salt and pepper

1 tablespoon (15 ml) ghee or duck fat

2–4 tablespoons (30–60 ml) water

Preheat the oven to 400°F (200°C) forced fan or 425°F (220°C) conventional.

Slice the cauliflower florets and place in a baking dish. Drizzle about ½ cup (120 ml) salsa verde over the cauliflower and set aside.

Pat the chicken thighs dry with a paper towel, and season with salt and pepper. Heat a large skillet greased with the ghee. Once hot, add the chicken thighs, skin-side down, and cook in batches for about 5 minutes, or until the skin is golden and crispy. Turn on the other side and cook for just 1 minute.

Place the cauliflower in the oven and bake for 5 minutes. After 5 minutes, place the chicken on top of the cauliflower in the baking dish, skin-side up. Deglaze the skillet by pouring the water into it, then pour the contents of the skillet over the cauliflower in the tray.

Bake for 20 to 25 minutes, tossing halfway through. The chicken is done when an instant-read thermometer inserted into the thickest part of the thigh reads 165°F (75°C).

Remove from the oven and drizzle with the remaining ½ cup (120 ml) salsa verde. Crispy chicken thighs are best served immediately. To store, let the chicken and vegetables cool, then store in the fridge for up to 4 days.

NUTRITION FACTS PER SERVING:
Total carbs: 9.2 g / Fiber: 3.6 g / Net carbs: 5.6 g / Protein: 30.9 g / Fat: 56.3 g / Calories: 590 kcal
Macronutrient ratio: Calories from carbs (3%), protein (19%), fat (78%)

Chicken Crust Meatza

SERVINGS: 4
HANDS-ON TIME: 10 minutes
OVERALL TIME: 40 minutes

This meatza is not what you might expect: The base is made in a similar way to jerky and the shredded mozzarella improves both the flavor and the texture of the crust. Serve with a green salad—one slice as a light lunch and two slices for a satisfying dinner.

CRUST BASE

1.1 pounds (500 g) ground chicken or turkey
½ teaspoon salt
¼ teaspoon black pepper
1½ cups (170 g/6 oz) shredded mozzarella

TOPPING

⅓ cup (80 ml) Marinara (page 55) or any sugar-free marinara/pizza sauce
4 ounces (115 g) frozen spinach, thawed and squeezed dry (weight excludes water squeezed out)
6 ounces (170 g) fresh mozzarella, sliced
¼ cup (60 ml) extra-virgin olive oil

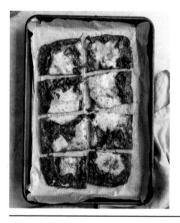

Preheat the oven to 400°F (200°C) forced fan or 425°F (220°C) conventional. Line a baking tray with parchment paper.

TO MAKE THE CRUST BASE: Place the ground meat in a food processor and add the salt, pepper, and mozzarella. Pulse to combine. Place the meaty mixture on the baking tray. Using your hands, flatten to create a large base, about ¼ inch (½ cm) thick. Place in the oven and bake for 25 to 30 minutes.

Remove from the oven and pour any excess juices out. Carefully flip onto the other side by placing another piece of parchment on top. Bake for 10 to 15 minutes. The aim is to get the crust crispy and free of excess moisture, just like jerky!

Flip one more time, spread the marinara on top, and add the spinach and mozzarella. Bake for 5 minutes, until the mozzarella is melted. To serve, drizzle with olive oil. Eat warm or store in the fridge for up to 4 days.

TIP:

Swap the ground chicken for turkey, beef, or even lamb. The leaner the meat, the better—the fats will cook out and you'll have less moisture to deal with.

NUTRITION FACTS PER SERVING (2 SLICES/¼ PIZZA):
Total carbs: 6 g / Fiber: 1.1 g / Net carbs: 4.9 g / Protein: 48.2 g / Fat: 35.3 g / Calories: 537 kcal
Macronutrient ratio: Calories from carbs (4%), protein (36%), fat (60%)

Lemon & Herb Chicken Tray Bake

SERVINGS: 4
HANDS-ON TIME: 15 minutes
OVERALL TIME: 35 minutes

   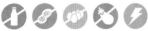

An easy sheet-pan bake made with Mediterranean herbs, zingy lemon, fragrant garlic, crispy chicken thighs, and low-carb veggies.

7.1 ounces (200 g) white mushrooms, sliced

14.1 ounces (400 g) green beans, trimmed

4 large or 8 small (900 g/2 lb.) bone-in chicken thighs

Pinch of salt and pepper

¼ cup (60 ml) ghee, duck fat, or olive oil, divided

2 tablespoons (30 ml) fresh lemon juice

¼ cup (60 ml) water or chicken stock

2 tablespoons (8 g/0.3 oz) chopped herbs (parsley, tarragon, thyme, and/or rosemary)

1 clove garlic, crushed

Preheat the oven to 400°F (200°C) forced fan or 425°F (220°C) conventional. Place the vegetables in a baking dish and set aside.

Pat the chicken thighs dry with a paper towel, and season with salt and pepper. Heat a large skillet greased with 2 tablespoons (30 ml) of ghee. Once hot, add the chicken thighs, skin-side down, and cook in batches for about 5 minutes, or until the skin is golden and crispy. Turn on the other side and cook for just 1 minute.

Place the chicken on top of the veggies in the baking dish, skin-side up. Deglaze the skillet by pouring the lemon juice and water into it, then pour over the veggies in the tray. Bake for 15 to 20 minutes, tossing halfway through the cooking time.

In a small bowl, mix the remaining 2 tablespoons (30 ml) ghee, herbs, and garlic. Drizzle over the chicken and the veggies, and place back in the oven for another 5 to 10 minutes. The chicken is done when an instant-read thermometer inserted into the thickest part of the thigh reads 165°F (75°C).

Crispy chicken thighs are best served immediately, optionally with more fresh herbs. To store, let the chicken and vegetables cool, then store in the fridge for up to 4 days.

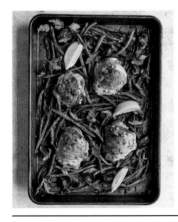

NUTRITION FACTS PER SERVING:
Total carbs: 9.4 g / Fiber: 3.3 g / Net carbs: 6.1 g / Protein: 30.2 g / Fat: 40.2 g / Calories: 510 kcal
Macronutrient ratio: Calories from carbs (5%), protein (24%), fat (71%)

Italian Melt Skillet

SERVINGS: 2
HANDS-ON TIME: 10 minutes
OVERALL TIME: 20 minutes

Juicy chicken topped with melty mozzarella and homemade marinara. This easy low-carb dish for two can be made in just twenty minutes. I like to serve mine with zoodles or a big bowl of crispy green salad.

1 large (250 g / 8.8 oz) chicken breast, skinless and boneless

Pinch of salt and pepper

1 tablespoon (15 ml) ghee or duck fat

⅓ cup (80 ml) Marinara (page 55) or any sugar-free marinara/pizza sauce

10 pitted olives (40 g / 1.4 oz), sliced

½ cup (57 g / 2 oz) shredded mozzarella

4 tablespoons (20 g / 0.7 oz) grated Parmesan

1 tablespoon (15 ml) extra-virgin olive oil

Fresh herbs, such as basil, parsley or thyme

Suggested side: steamed greens, lemon juice, and olive oil; zucchini noodles (page 34), raw or briefly cooked with more marinara sauce

To butterfly the chicken breast, place it on a chopping board. Placing your hand flat on top of the chicken breast, use a sharp knife to slice into one side, starting at the thicker end and ending at the thinner point. Be careful not to cut all the way through to the other side. Open the breast so that it resembles a butterfly, about ½ inch (1 cm) thick. Season with salt and pepper.

Heat a large skillet greased with ghee over medium-high heat. Once hot, add the butterflied chicken. Cook undisturbed for 5 to 7 minutes. Rotate the pan halfway through to ensure even cooking. Then flip the chicken over and cook for 1 minute. Top with marinara, olives, mozzarella, and Parmesan. Place under a broiler for 2 to 3 minutes, until the cheese is melted and lightly crisped up. Drizzle with the olive oil, and sprinkle with fresh herbs. Serve with steamed greens drizzled with lemon and olive oil, or zucchini noodles with more marinara. Store in the fridge for up to 4 days.

NUTRITION FACTS PER SERVING:
Total carbs: 5 g / Fiber: 1.2 g / Net carbs: 3.8 g / Protein: 39.2 g / Fat: 27.6 g / Calories: 430 kcal
Macronutrient ratio: Calories from carbs (4%), protein (37%), fat (59%)

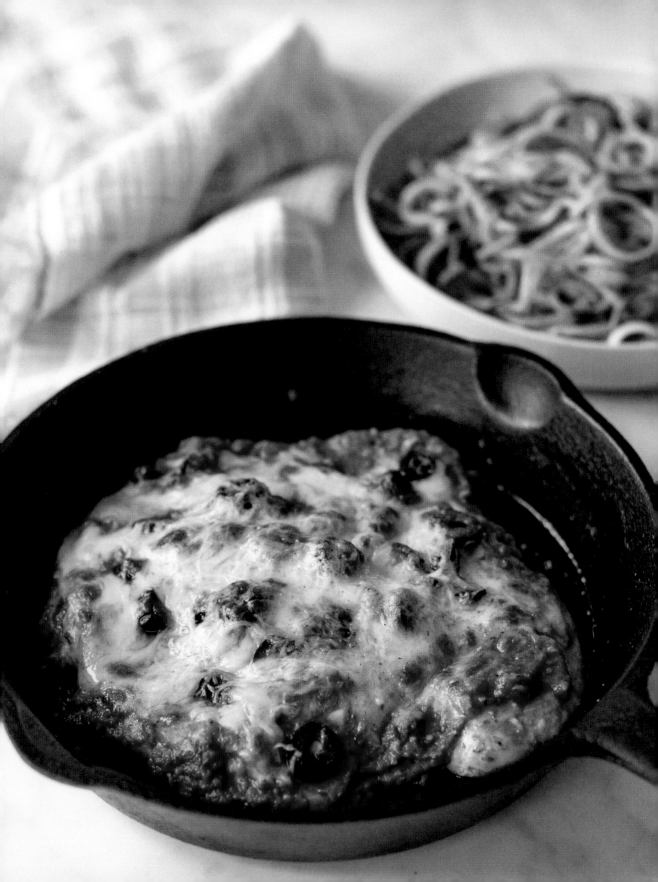

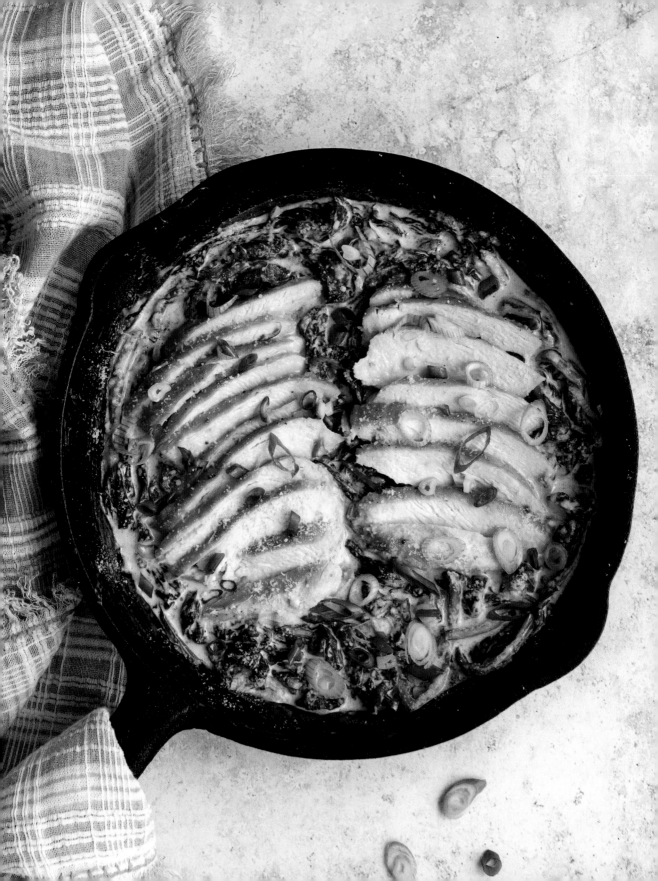

Creamed Spinach Chicken Skillet

SERVINGS: 2
HANDS-ON TIME: 15 minutes
OVERALL TIME: 20 minutes

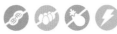

Creamed spinach is the perfect keto side. Simply top with cooked chicken and you've got a delicious one-pot meal in just twenty minutes. This recipe makes two servings so you can have one for dinner and pack the rest for the next day's lunch!

1 tablespoon (15 ml) ghee or duck fat

2 medium (300 g/10.6 oz) chicken breasts, skinless and boneless (150 g/5.3 oz each)

½ cup (120 ml) heavy whipping cream

10.6 ounces (300 g) frozen spinach, thawed and squeezed dry (weight excludes water squeezed out)

Optional: pinch of nutmeg

Pinch of salt and pepper

4 tablespoons (20 g/0.8 oz) grated Parmesan cheese, divided

1 medium (15 g/0.5 oz) spring onion, sliced

Optional: fresh herbs of choice

Heat a large skillet greased with ghee over medium-high heat. Once hot, add the chicken, skin-side down. Cook undisturbed for 5 to 8 minutes. Rotate the pan halfway through to ensure even cooking. Then flip the chicken over and cook for another 5 to 8 minutes. The exact time depends on the thickness. The chicken is done when an instant-read thermometer inserted into the thickest part of the breast reads 165°F (75°C). Remove from the pan and place on a chopping board. Leave to cool slightly and then slice.

Place the cream in the pan where you cooked the chicken. Add the drained spinach. Add a pinch of nutmeg (if using), salt, and pepper. Gently heat until it begins to simmer and cook to thicken for 1 minute. Then mix in 3 tablespoons (15 g/0.5 oz) of the Parmesan. Top with the sliced cooked chicken breasts and sprinkle with the remaining 1 tablespoon (5 g) Parmesan. Serve warm sprinkled with the spring onion or herbs of choice. Store in the fridge for up to 4 days.

TIP:
Instead of ½ cup (120 ml) heavy whipping cream you can use ¼ cup (60 g/2.1 oz) mascarpone or full-fat cream cheese.

NUTRITION FACTS PER SERVING:
Total carbs: 8.8 g / Fiber: 4.5 g / Net carbs: 4.3 g / Protein: 44.1 g / Fat: 37.7 g / Calories: 553 kcal
Macronutrient ratio: Calories from carbs (3%), protein (33%), fat (64%)

Duck Breasts with Cabbage Noodles

SERVINGS: 2
HANDS-ON TIME: 15 minutes
OVERALL TIME: 30 minutes

This is my favorite way to eat duck breasts—super simple with buttery lemon cabbage noodles. This meal is ultra-low in carbs and full of flavor!

2 duck breasts (340 g/ 12 oz total), skin on
Pinch of salt and pepper
2 tablespoons (30 ml) ghee or duck fat
¼ medium (300 g/ 10.6 oz) green cabbage, sliced into wide "noodles"
1 tablespoon (15 ml) fresh lemon juice
2–4 tablespoons (30–60 ml) water
Optional: crispy bacon added to the cooked cabbage

Preheat the oven to 430°F (220°C) forced fan or 465°F (240°C) conventional. Score the skin on the duck breasts, and season with salt and pepper.

Heat a medium pan over medium-high heat. Place the duck breasts skin-side down in the hot dry pan (no oil needed) and reduce the heat. As the duck fat is released, use a spoon to baste the breasts with it regularly, and cook for 6 to 8 minutes, or until lightly golden. Flip over and cook for about 30 seconds, just to "seal" them on the other side.

Place the duck breasts skin-side up in a baking tray and bake for 10 minutes (rare), 15 minutes (medium), or 18 minutes (well done). Let the duck breasts rest on a cooling rack for 10 minutes before slicing and serving.

To the pan where you cooked the duck, add the ghee and the cabbage. Toss to combine. Add the lemon juice and water and cover with a lid. Cook over medium-low heat for 3 to 5 minutes. Remove the lid and cook for another 3 to 5 minutes. Optionally, crumble the bacon on the cabbage, and serve with the duck breasts. Duck breasts are best served while still warm, but they can be refrigerated in a sealed container for up to 4 days.

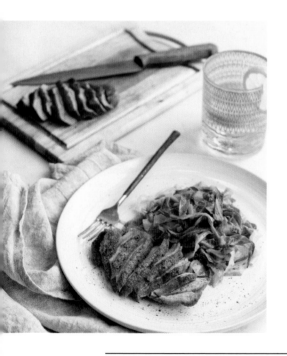

NUTRITION FACTS PER SERVING:
Total carbs: 9.1 g / Fiber: 3.8 g / Net carbs: 5.3 g / Protein: 31.1 g / Fat: 41 g / Calories: 526 kcal
Macronutrient ratio: Calories from carbs (4%), protein (24%), fat (72%)

Tandoori Beef Skillet

SERVINGS: 2
HANDS-ON TIME: 15 minutes
OVERALL TIME: 20 minutes

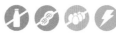

An easy one-pot dinner for two infused with Indian spices. Feel free to swap the cauliflower for other veggies. Chopped broccoli or zucchini work best!

1 teaspoon ghee or duck fat

10.6 ounces (300 g) ground beef

1½ teaspoons onion powder

½ teaspoon garlic powder

2 teaspoons (4 g) tandoori spice mix

Salt and pepper, to taste

½ medium (300 g/10.6 oz) cauliflower, chopped

2 tablespoons (30 ml) water

¼ cup (60 ml) coconut cream or heavy whipping cream

Fresh herbs, such as parsley or cilantro

Heat a medium skillet greased with ghee over high heat. Add the beef, onion powder, garlic powder, tandoori spice, and a pinch of salt and pepper. Cook for 2 minutes, stirring frequently. Add the cauliflower, water, and coconut cream.

Bring to a boil and then reduce the heat to medium-low and cover with a lid. Cook for about 8 minutes. Remove the lid and cook for another 2 to 3 minutes, until the cauliflower is crisp-tender and the excess juices evaporate. Season to taste.

Eat warm, sprinkled with fresh herbs to taste. To store, refrigerate for up to 4 days.

TIP:

If tandoori spice mix is too spicy for you, swap it for mild curry powder or garam masala.

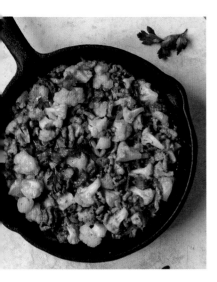

NUTRITION FACTS PER SERVING:
Total carbs: 12.1 g / Fiber: 4.4 g / Net carbs: 7.7 g / Protein: 30.1 g / Fat: 43.4 g / Calories: 552 kcal
Macronutrient ratio: Calories from carbs (6%), protein (22%), fat (72%)

Classic "Naked" Burgers

SERVINGS: 2
HANDS-ON TIME: 15 minutes
OVERALL TIME: 20 minutes

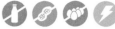

Naked burgers, skinny burgers, or bunless burgers are all names for burgers that are served without the bread rolls. These burgers are better than your regular take-out meal! It's easy to scale up or down, so you can make as many burgers as you need. The serving size is generous, so feel free to make smaller burgers if you prefer.

BURGERS

12 ounces (340 g) ground beef
1 teaspoon onion powder
¼ teaspoon garlic powder
½ teaspoon apple cider vinegar
Generous pinch of salt and pepper
1 teaspoon ghee or duck fat for greasing
Optional: 2 slices (50 g/1.8 oz) American, Cheddar, or provolone cheese

SAUCE

2 tablespoons (30 g/1.1 oz) mayonnaise (page 16)
2 teaspoons (10 g/0.4 oz) tomato paste
1 teaspoon fresh lemon juice or pickle juice
1 teaspoon chopped fresh herbs of choice (basil, parsley, dill, or chives), or 1–2 teaspoons grated pickle
Salt and pepper, to taste

TO ASSEMBLE

1 head green lettuce, crispy large outer leaves only, core removed (200 g/7.1 oz), iceberg works best
4 slices (120 g/4.2 oz) medium tomato
4 slices (20 g/0.7 oz) medium red onion
1 small (20 g/0.7 oz) pickle, sliced

TO MAKE THE BURGERS: Combine the beef, onion powder, garlic powder, vinegar, salt, and pepper in a bowl. Divide the ground meat in 2 equal parts. Use your hands to shape each piece into a loose burger, about 4½ inches (12 cm) in diameter and ½ to ¾ inch (1¼ to 2 cm) thick. Pierce the patties with a fork several times. This will loosen the patties and help them cook evenly without curling or getting tough while enabling maximum caramelization.

Heat a large pan greased with the ghee over high heat. Use a spatula to transfer the burgers to the hot pan. Cook for 2 to 3 minutes, then flip over with the spatula, and cook for an additional 2 to 3 minutes. If using cheese, place it on top of the burgers for the last minute of the cooking process. Set aside.

TO MAKE THE SAUCE: Mix the mayo, tomato paste, lemon juice, and herbs in a bowl. Season with salt and pepper.

TO ASSEMBLE THE BURGERS: Halve the lettuce and remove the middle part; you should end up with a crispy lettuce shell made of 2 to 3 layers of outer leaves. Place the burger inside the shell and top with the tomatoes, onion, pickles, and the prepared burger sauce. Eat while still warm.

TIPS:
• Are you dairy-free? Swap the cheese for crispy bacon slices or a panfried egg with runny yolk.
• Are you egg-free? Swap the mayo for crème fraîche or sour cream.

PICTURED ON PAGE 111

NUTRITION FACTS PER SERVING (1 BURGER):
Total carbs: 9.8 g / Fiber: 2.8 g / Net carbs: 7 g / Protein: 37.6 g / Fat: 57.7 g / Calories: 709 kcal
Macronutrient ratio: Calories from carbs (4%), protein (22%), fat (74%)

Lemon & Herb Steak with Green Beans

SERVINGS: 1
HANDS-ON TIME: 10 minutes
OVERALL TIME: 20 minutes

Enjoy this single-serve steak dish with herby lemon sauce and green beans for a healthy dinner in just twenty minutes!

1 medium (150 g/5.3 oz) sirloin, rump, or fillet steak

Pinch of salt and pepper

1 tablespoon (15 ml) ghee or duck fat

1 tablespoon (14 g/0.5 oz) butter, ghee, or olive oil

1½ teaspoons fresh lemon juice

1 tablespoon (4 g/0.2 oz) chopped parsley or herbs of choice

5.3 ounces (150 g) fresh or frozen green beans, trimmed

Optional: lemon wedges

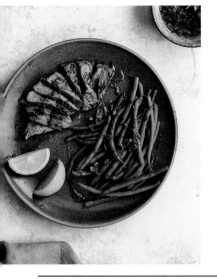

Allow the steak to sit at room temperature for a few minutes. Using a paper towel, pat off the excess moisture. Season with salt and pepper. Fry in a very hot, heavy-bottomed pan greased with ghee over high heat for 2 to 4 minutes on each side to let the meat caramelize and seal in the juices. When you see the sides getting brown, it's time to flip it over. Reduce to medium heat and continue to cook for 4 minutes (rare), 7 minutes (medium), or 11 minutes (well done). Remove the steak from the pan and allow it to rest in a warm place for 5 to 7 minutes. The steak will finish cooking in the residual heat as the temperature slowly goes down.

Meanwhile, deglaze the hot pan where you cooked the steak by adding the butter, lemon juice, and herbs. Pour into a small bowl and keep warm.

In a saucepan, bring about 1 cup (240 ml) of water to a boil. Put the green beans in a steamer basket, set it over the boiling water inside the saucepan, cover, and steam for 3 to 5 minutes, until tender to the bite. Serve the green beans immediately with the steak and drizzled with the sauce. Optionally, serve with lemon wedges.

TIPS:

• You can swap the sirloin for skirt steak, flank steak, or fatty cuts such as rib eye.

• Need to reduce the carb count? Swap the green beans for asparagus or spinach! Instead of steaming you can pan-roast the green beans for extra caramelized flavor. To do that, simply place the green beans in a hot pan greased with ghee or olive oil. Cook for 5 to 7 minutes, until they are blistering and browning. Season with salt and pepper, add water, reduce the heat to medium, and cover with a lid. Cook, covered, for 1 to 2 minutes, until the beans are bright green and crisp-tender.

NUTRITION FACTS PER SERVING:
Total carbs: 11.2 g / Fiber: 4.2 g / Net carbs: 7 g / Protein: 34.1 g / Fat: 43.5 g / Calories: 571 kcal
Macronutrient ratio: Calories from carbs (5%), protein (25%), fat (70%)

Alfredo Meatball Pasta

SERVINGS: 4
HANDS-ON TIME: 20 minutes
OVERALL TIME: 30 minutes

This easy low-carb dish is everything that is good in the world of comfort foods. Creamy, cheesy sauce, slurpy zero-carb noodles with nutrient-dense kale, crowned with juicy beef meatballs. It's ideal if you have higher energy needs and for breaking your fasting window!

¼ cup (57g/2 oz) unsalted butter

¾ cup (180 ml) heavy whipping cream

½ teaspoon garlic powder

Pinch of salt and pepper

⅔ cup (60g/2.1 oz) grated Parmesan

1.1 pounds (500 g) ground beef

2 teaspoons (2 g/0.1 oz) dried Italian herbs or 2 tablespoons (8 g/0.3 oz) fresh chopped herbs

1 clove garlic, minced

1 large egg

3 tablespoons (24 g/0.9 oz) coconut flour or ½ cup (50 g/1.8 oz) almond flour

Pinch of salt and pepper

1 tablespoon (15 ml) ghee or duck fat, for frying

7.1 ounces (200 g) chopped kale, stems removed, or spinach

¼ cup (60 ml) water

3 packs (300 g/10.6 oz total) shirataki noodles or shirataki fettucine, prepared according to instructions on page 14

To make the sauce, add the butter and heavy whipping cream to a large saucepan over low heat. Simmer, stirring, for 3 minutes. Whisk in garlic powder, salt, pepper, and then grated Parmesan. Cook until melted and slightly thickened. Set aside and keep warm. Place the beef, herbs, garlic, egg, coconut flour, and a generous pinch of salt and pepper in a mixing bowl. Mix until well combined. Using your hands, create 20 meatballs (about 29 g/1 oz each) from the mixture.

Grease a large pan with ghee and place it over medium heat. When hot, add the meatballs in a single layer. Cook for 2 minutes on each side, turning with a fork until browned on all sides and cooked through. Transfer the meatballs to a plate and keep warm.

To the pan where you cooked the meatballs, add the kale. Cook for 1 to 2 minutes, tossing well. Add the water and cover with a lid. Cook for 3 to 5 minutes, until tender. If using spinach, do not add any water and cook uncovered for 1 minute, until wilted.

Add the prepared shirataki noodles and pour in the Alfredo sauce. Toss to combine and season to taste. Return the meatballs to the pan and cook briefly to warm through. Serve warm. Store in the fridge for up to 4 days.

TIP:

Alfredo sauce can also be served drizzled over veggies or meat. If not serving straight away, store the sauce in the fridge for up to 4 days. Reheat over low heat, whisking to combine and avoid separation, or give the sauce a quick blitz using a hand blender. This recipe makes about 1¼ cups/300 ml sauce and can be easily scaled up or down.

NUTRITION FACTS PER SERVING (5 MEATBALLS + VEG, NOODLES & SAUCE):
Total carbs: 9.4 g / Fiber: 3.4 g / Net carbs: 6 g / Protein: 31.5 g / Fat: 63.7 g / Calories: 737 kcal
Macronutrient ratio: Calories from carbs (3%), protein (17%), fat (80%)

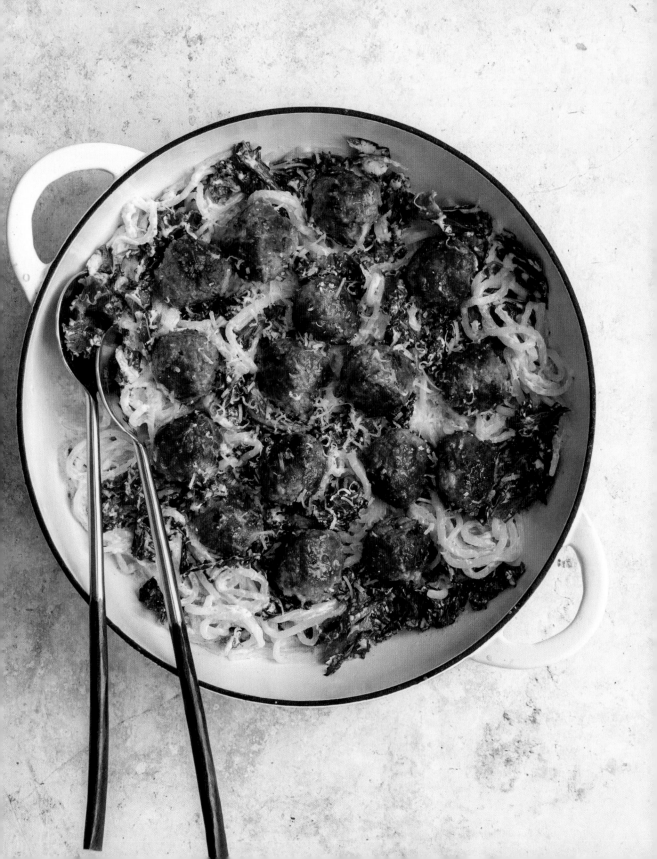

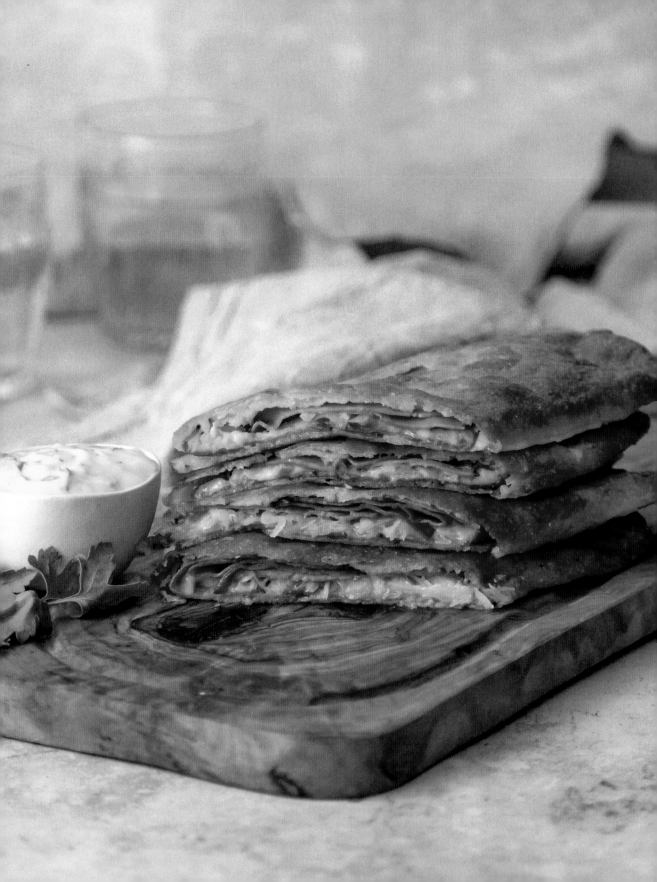

Reuben Hot Pockets

SERVINGS: 2
HANDS-ON TIME: 15 minutes
OVERALL TIME: 30 minutes

I must make a dozen recipes using this super simple keto dough! It's so versatile and can be filled with anything sweet and savory. Here's my favorite recipe with sauerkraut, pastrami, and Swiss cheese.

DOUGH
¾ cup (85 g/3 oz) shredded mozzarella
⅓ cup (33 g/1.2 oz) almond flour

FILLING
3 ounces (85 g) sliced pastrami or
 quality ham
3 ounces (85 g) sliced Swiss cheese
¼ cup (36 g/1.3 oz) drained sauerkraut

Prepare the dough by melting the mozzarella in the microwave for about 1 minute. Alternatively, you can melt the cheese in the oven at 300°F (150°C) forced fan or 340°F (170°C) conventional for 5 to 10 minutes. Mix and add the almond flour. Stir until well combined.

Preheat or increase the temperature of the oven to 355°F (180°C) forced fan or 400°F (200°C) conventional.

Roll out the dough thinly between 2 sheets of parchment paper or use a nonstick mat and nonstick rolling pin. When rolled out, the dough should be about 8 x 11 inches (20 x 30 cm).

Add the pastrami followed by the cheese and drained sauerkraut to the center of the dough, then fold over like an envelope and seal the dough with your fingers. Using a sharp knife, poke some holes into the dough to release the steam while baking. Bake for 15 to 20 minutes, until golden brown.

Serve warm with mayonnaise (page 16), or store in a sealed container and refrigerate for up to 4 days.

TIPS:
• Are you nut-free? You can easily convert this recipe by adding 2 ounces (57 g) of full-fat cream cheese to the shredded mozzarella before microwaving it, and then swapping the almond flour for either 6 tablespoons (48 g/1.7 oz) of coconut flour or 8 tablespoons (57 g/2 oz) of flax meal.

• Instead of mayo, you can serve these with a spicy horseradish dressing made with 3 tablespoons (45 g/1.5 oz) mayonnaise (page 16), 1 tablespoon (15 g/0.5 oz) sour cream or more mayo, 1 teaspoon sriracha sauce or tomato paste, 1 tablespoon (15 ml) fresh lemon juice, 2 tablespoons (8 g/0.3 oz) sliced spring onions, chives, or parsley, ½ teaspoon prepared horseradish, 1 small (15 g/0.5 oz) grated pickle, salt, and pepper to taste.

NUTRITION FACTS PER SERVING (½ POCKET):
Total carbs: 7.1 g / Fiber: 2.4 g / Net carbs: 4.7 g / Protein: 37.2 g / Fat: 31.7 g / Calories: 456 kcal
Macronutrient ratio: Calories from carbs (4%), protein (33%), fat (63%)

Skillet Shepherd's Pie

SERVINGS: 5
HANDS-ON TIME: 30 minutes
OVERALL TIME: 1 hour

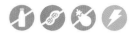

This shepherd's pie is the ultimate keto comfort food. I was told by my British friends that it's better than the traditional recipe. All I can say is that it's a staple in my house! It's packed with flavor from herbs and spices and it's super creamy thanks to egg yolks that act as a thickener and make a fantastic grain-free gravy. My favorite part is the cheesy cauli-mash topping broiled to perfection!

1 recipe Cheesy Cauli-Mash (page 66), grated Cheddar reserved for topping

1 tablespoon (15 ml) ghee or duck fat

½ small (35 g/1.2 oz) yellow onion, diced

2 cloves garlic, minced

1.3 pounds (600 g) ground beef

1 tablespoon (15 ml) apple cider vinegar

1 teaspoon dried herbs (oregano, thyme, or rosemary)

1 teaspoon cumin powder

Optional: ⅛ teaspoon cayenne pepper for extra heat

Generous pinch of salt and pepper

½ medium (60 g/2.1 oz) red bell pepper, diced

1 cup (100 g/3.5 oz) chopped green beans

4 egg yolks

½ cup (120 ml) chicken stock, bone broth, or water

Prepare the cauli-mash according to instructions on page 66 and reserve all the grated Cheddar for topping.

Heat a large ovenproof skillet greased with ghee over medium-high heat. Any deep skillet that is at least 10 inches (25 cm) in diameter will work. Add the onion and cook for 5 minutes. Add the garlic, beef, vinegar, herbs, cumin, optional cayenne pepper, salt, and pepper. Cook until opaque while stirring for 3 to 5 minutes. Add the bell pepper and green beans. Cover the skillet with a lid, reduce the heat to medium, and cook for about 8 minutes.

Preheat the oven to 430°F (220°C) forced fan or 465°F (240°C) conventional.

In a bowl, whisk the egg yolks with the stock. Increase the heat to medium-high, pour the egg yolk mixture into the skillet, and cook while stirring constantly until the sauce thickens. Take off the heat and add the cheesy cauli-mash, leaving about a 1-inch (2.5 cm) gap between the edges of the pan and the cauli-mash. This will allow the excess juices from the meaty layer to escape.

Sprinkle the reserved ½ cup (57 g/2 oz) Cheddar on top. Place in the preheated oven and bake for 15 to 20 minutes, until the top is golden and crisp.

TIPS:
• Feel free to swap the beef for ground lamb.
• Are you dairy-free? Swap the Cheesy Cauli-Mash for the Caramelized Onion Cauli-Mash (page 66).

PICTURED ON PAGE 111

NUTRITION FACTS PER SERVING (⅕ PIE):
Total carbs: 11.3 g / Fiber: 3.6 g / Net carbs: 7.7 g / Protein: 30.4 g / Fat: 52.9 g / Calories: 632 kcal
Macronutrient ratio: Calories from carbs (5%), protein (19%), fat (76%)

Marinated Pork Belly Tray Bake

SERVINGS: 4
HANDS-ON TIME: 10 minutes
OVERALL TIME: 1 hour 30 minutes

Pork belly is perfect for a keto diet. It's basically a thick cut of uncured and unsalted bacon, and you won't need to add any fats to cook. When combined with spices and meat juices, it makes the most amazing sauce to cook your veg!

RUB

1 tablespoon (7 g/0.3 oz) paprika

½ teaspoon onion powder

¼ teaspoon garlic powder

1 tablespoon (2 g/0.1 oz) dried marjoram or oregano

½ teaspoon black pepper

½ teaspoon salt

Optional: 1 teaspoon erythritol or Swerve

TRAY BAKE

1.1 pounds (500 g) pork belly

1 tablespoon (15 ml) apple cider vinegar

¼ cup (60 ml) water

1.3 pounds (600 g) asparagus, trimmed

TO MAKE THE SPICE RUB: Combine all the ingredients in a small bowl.

TO MAKE THE TRAY BAKE: Slice the pork belly into 8 slices, about ½ inch (1 cm) each. Place the pork belly slices on a tray and brush with the vinegar. Sprinkle with the spice rub on all sides, making sure that all slices are covered. Place in the fridge and marinate for at least 30 minutes or overnight.

Preheat the oven to 400°F (200°C) forced fan or 425°F (220°C) conventional.

Place the slices side by side in a baking dish. Add the water, cover with aluminum foil, and bake for 25 to 30 minutes. Remove from the oven and transfer the pork belly slices to a large plate.

Reduce the temperature to 350°F (175°C) forced fan or 380°F (195°C) conventional. Add the asparagus to the tray and toss to cover in the rendered fat and juices. Add back the pork belly slices, crispy-side down, and place back in the oven. Bake for 8 to 12 minutes, until the asparagus is crisp-tender.

Serve warm. Store in the fridge for up to 4 days.

TIP:

This meal is very high in fat and relatively low in protein. To reduce the fat content, you can pour some of the rendered lard into a jar and use for cooking, or discard. Alternatively, swap half of the pork belly for lean pork chops. Doing that will also increase the protein content.

NUTRITION FACTS PER SERVING (2 SLICES + ASPARAGUS):
Total carbs: 7.6 g / Fiber: 4.1 g / Net carbs: 3.5 g / Protein: 15.4 g / Fat: 66.7 g / Calories: 687 kcal
Macronutrient ratio: Calories from carbs (2%), protein (9%), fat (89%)

Sheet-Pan Lemon & Garlic Pork Chops

SERVINGS: 4
HANDS-ON TIME: 10 minutes
OVERALL TIME: 40 minutes

These low-carb, sheet-pan pork chops are ideal for busy weeknights. It's a great way to get speedy family-friendly dinner ready in under an hour with minimum washing up to do.

4 large (680 g/1.5) boneless pork chops (about 170 g/6 oz each)

Pinch of salt and pepper

4 tablespoons (60 ml) ghee, duck fat, olive oil, or avocado oil, divided

1.1 pounds (500 g) Brussels sprouts, halved

2 tablespoons (30 ml) fresh lemon juice

¼ cup (60 ml) water

2 cloves garlic, crushed

1 tablespoon (4 g/0.2 oz) chopped thyme or 1 teaspoon dried thyme

Preheat the oven to 400°F (200°C) forced fan or 425°F (220°C) conventional.

Season the pork chops with salt and pepper. Heat a large pan greased with 1 tablespoon (15 ml) of ghee over high heat. Fry the pork chops in batches for 1 to 2 minutes per side. Transfer to a baking dish, add the Brussels sprouts, and set aside.

Deglaze the pan with the lemon juice and water and pour over the pork chops and Brussels sprouts. Bake for 25 to 30 minutes, rotating the tray halfway to ensure even cooking.

Meanwhile, mix the remaining 3 tablespoons (45 ml) ghee, garlic, and thyme in a bowl. Brush over the pork chops and Brussels sprouts, return to the oven, and bake for another 5 minutes.

Serve warm or store in the fridge for up to 4 days.

TIP:

Need to reduce the carb count? Swap the Brussels sprouts for asparagus or green beans. Add them in the last 15 minutes of baking to avoid overcooking.

NUTRITION FACTS PER SERVING:
Total carbs: 12.2 g / Fiber: 4.8 g / Net carbs: 7.4 g / Protein: 39.2 g / Fat: 30.6 g / Calories: 480 kcal
Macronutrient ratio: Calories from carbs (6%), protein (34%), fat (60%)

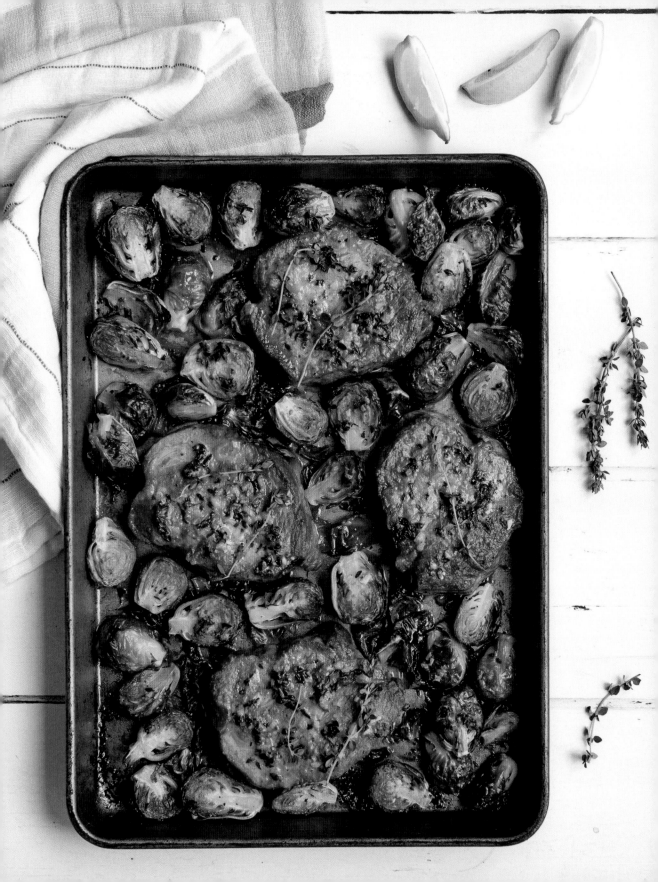

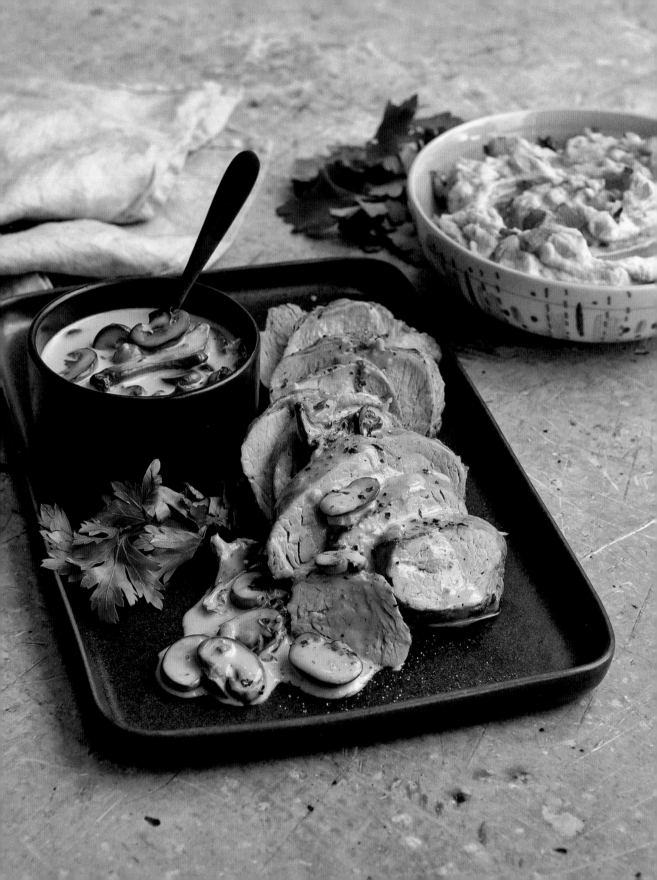

Pork Tenderloin with Creamy Mushroom Gravy

SERVINGS: 4
HANDS-ON TIME: 20 minutes
OVERALL TIME: 35 minutes

Pork tenderloin is naturally lean and ideal to pair with high-fat creamy mushroom sauce. This is best served with cauli-rice, sautéed greens, or steamed low-carb veggies such as green beans or asparagus.

1 pound (450 g) pork tenderloin

Pinch of salt and pepper

3 tablespoons (45 ml) ghee, duck fat, olive oil, or avocado oil, divided

2 cloves garlic, minced

1½ cups (115 g/4 oz) sliced brown mushrooms or mixed wild mushrooms

½ cup (120 ml) chicken stock or water

1 tablespoon (15 ml) fresh lemon juice

¾ cup (180 ml) heavy whipping cream

Suggested sides: Caramelized Onion Cauli-Mash (page 66) and steamed green beans, asparagus, broccoli, or more roasted mushrooms

Preheat the oven to 375°F (190°C) forced fan or 410°F (210°C) conventional.

Pat the tenderloin dry with a paper towel, and season with salt and pepper. Heat a large ovenproof skillet greased with 1 tablespoon (15 ml) of ghee over high heat. Add the tenderloin and cook until browned on all sides, about 3 to 4 minutes. Place in a baking dish, transfer to the oven, and bake for about 20 minutes. When done, remove from the oven, cover with aluminum foil, and place on a cooling rack.

While the tenderloin is baking, prepare the creamy mushroom sauce: Add the remaining 2 tablespoons (30 ml) of ghee to the skillet where you browned the tenderloin. Add the garlic and mushrooms and cook over medium-high heat for about 5 minutes. Add the stock and lemon juice. Bring to a boil and cook for another 2 to 3 minutes, until the mushrooms are tender. Add the cream, bring to a boil, and cook to thicken slightly. Take off the heat and season to taste.

Serve the cooked sliced tenderloin warm with the sauce and a side dish of your choice. Refrigerate for up to 4 days.

NUTRITION FACTS PER SERVING (¼ TENDERLOIN + ABOUT ½ CUP SAUCE):
Total carbs: 3.2 g / Fiber: 0.2 g / Net carbs: 3 g / Protein: 25.7 g / Fat: 31.2 g / Calories: 404 kcal
Macronutrient ratio: Calories from carbs (3%), protein (26%), fat (71%)

Egg Roll in a Bowl

SERVINGS: 4
HANDS-ON TIME: 15 minutes
OVERALL TIME: 20 minutes

All the delicious flavors of your favorite Chinese appetizer in one healthy nutritious bowl. A tasty keto-friendly dinner in less than twenty minutes!

2 tablespoons (30 ml) ghee, duck fat, olive oil, or avocado oil

4 medium (60 g/2.1 oz) spring onions, sliced

2 cloves garlic, minced

1.1 pounds (500 g) ground pork (20% fat)

¼ cup (60 ml) coconut aminos or tamari sauce

1.1 pounds (500 g) coleslaw mix (you can use store-bought or make your own [page 71])

2 tablespoons (30 ml) fresh lime or lemon juice

Salt and pepper, to taste

Optional: 1 teaspoon toasted sesame oil, 2 teaspoons (6 g/0.2 oz) sesame seeds, and lime wedges

Heat a large skillet greased with ghee over medium-high heat. Add the white parts of the sliced spring onions and garlic. Cook for 1 minute. Add the ground pork and cook for about 5 minutes, until browned on all sides. Add the coconut aminos, coleslaw mix, and lime juice. Cook for 5 to 8 minutes, stirring frequently, until the veggies are wilted and the meat is cooked through. Take off the heat and season to taste.

Mix in the sliced green parts of the spring onions. Serve warm, optionally with toasted sesame oil, sesame seeds, and lime wedges. To store, refrigerate for up to 4 days.

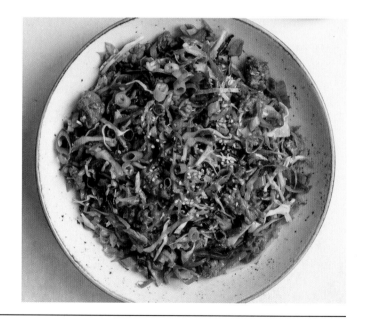

NUTRITION FACTS PER SERVING:
Total carbs: 10.3 g / Fiber: 3.4 g / Net carbs: 6.9 g / Protein: 23 g / Fat: 34 g / Calories: 439 kcal
Macronutrient ratio: Calories from carbs (6%), protein (22%), fat (72%)

Greek-Style Lamburger Stacks

SERVINGS: 2
HANDS-ON TIME: 20 minutes
OVERALL TIME: 25 minutes

None of my cookbooks would be complete without a satisfying Greek-inspired dish! These easy bunless burgers are made with lamb instead of beef and served between thick slices of grilled eggplant with refreshing, herby cucumber tzatziki dip.

TZATZIKI DIP

½ cup (120 g/4.2 oz) full-fat Greek yogurt
½ small (60 g/2.1 oz) cucumber, grated
½ clove garlic, crushed
½ tablespoon (2 g/0.1 oz) chopped dill or ½ teaspoon dried dill
2 teaspoons (10 ml) lemon juice, plus optionally ½ teaspoon fresh lemon zest
Salt and pepper, to taste

EGGPLANT

4 slices (300 g/10.6 oz) of the middle part of a large eggplant, each slice about 1 inch (2.5 cm) thick
2 tablespoons (30 ml) ghee or olive oil
Salt and pepper, to taste

LAMB PATTIES

12 ounces (340 g) ground lamb
Pinch of salt and pepper
1 teaspoon ghee or duck fat, for greasing
Optional: spinach, watercress, or beet greens

TO MAKE THE TZATZIKI: Combine all the ingredients in a bowl. Place in the fridge while you prepare the burgers.

TO MAKE THE EGGPLANT: Heat a large pan or a griddle pan over medium heat. Brush the eggplant slices with the ghee on both sides, and season with salt and pepper. Cook the slices for about 5 minutes on each side, until soft and browned. Remove from the pan and keep warm.

TO MAKE THE LAMB PATTIES: Gently divide the ground meat in 2 equal parts. Use your hands to shape each piece into a loose burger, 4½ inches (12 cm) in diameter and ½ to ¾ inch (1¼ to 2 cm) thick. Do not squeeze or pack the meat too tightly, or the burgers will lose their juiciness as they are cooked. Season with salt and pepper on each side.

Heat the pan where you cooked the eggplants over high heat and grease with 1 teaspoon of ghee. Use a spatula to transfer the burgers to the hot pan. Cook for 3 minutes, then flip over with the spatula, and cook for an additional 2 to 3 minutes.

Put each patty between 2 slices of the grilled eggplant. Serve with the prepared tzatziki and optionally with a big handful of crispy greens such as spinach, watercress, or beet greens.

TIP:

Swap the eggplant for 4 pan-roasted portobello mushrooms!

PICTURED ON PAGE 111

NUTRITION FACTS PER SERVING (1 LAMBURGER + ABOUT ⅓ CUP + 1 TABLESPOON TZATZIKI):
Total carbs: 12.5 g / Fiber: 4.8 g / Net carbs: 7.7 g / Protein: 36.5 g / Fat: 53.7 g / Calories: 673 kcal
Macronutrient ratio: Calories from carbs (5%), protein (22%), fat (73%)

Ground Shish Kebab with Cucumber Raita

SERVINGS: 4
HANDS-ON TIME: 25 minutes
OVERALL TIME: 25 minutes

I once made these lamb kebabs for a summer barbecue. I didn't follow any particular recipe but simply used my favorite spices. Everyone enjoyed it, including "keto skeptics"! Initially I planned to make these as meatballs, but we ended up cooking them on skewers because it's less fussy and requires minimum prep time.

CUCUMBER RAITA

1½ cups (375 g/13.2 oz) full-fat yogurt
1 small (150 g/5.3 oz) cucumber, grated
2 tablespoons (8 g/0.3 oz) chopped mint
1 tablespoon (15 ml) fresh lemon juice
½ teaspoon fresh lemon zest
½ teaspoon ground cumin
Salt and pepper, to taste

LAMB KEBABS

1.1 pounds (500 g) ground lamb
2 teaspoons (4 g/0.2 oz) ground cumin
2 teaspoons (5 g/0.2 oz) paprika
½ teaspoon onion powder
1 clove garlic, minced
1 tablespoon (15 ml) ghee
Optional: spinach, watercress, or beet greens

TO MAKE THE CUCUMBER RAITA: Combine all the ingredients in a bowl. Place in the fridge while you prepare the kebabs.

TO MAKE THE KEBABS: Place all the ingredients for the kebabs, except the ghee, in a bowl. Mix until well combined. Divide the meat mixture into 8 parts (about 64 g/2.3 oz each). Using your hands, form oval-shaped kebabs around each of 8 skewers.

Heat a griddle pan greased with the ghee over medium-high heat. Place the skewers in the pan in a single layer and cook for 5 to 7 minutes, turning frequently, until browned on all sides and cooked through.

Serve with the cucumber raita and optionally with a big handful of crispy greens such as spinach, watercress, or beet greens. Store in the fridge in two separate containers for up to 4 days.

NUTRITION FACTS PER SERVING (2 KEBABS + ABOUT ⅔ CUP CUCUMBER RAITA):
Total carbs: 6.6 g / Fiber: 1 g / Net carbs: 5.5 g / Protein: 30.6 g / Fat: 34.8 g / Calories: 459 kcal
Macronutrient ratio: Calories from carbs (5%), protein (27%), fat (68%)

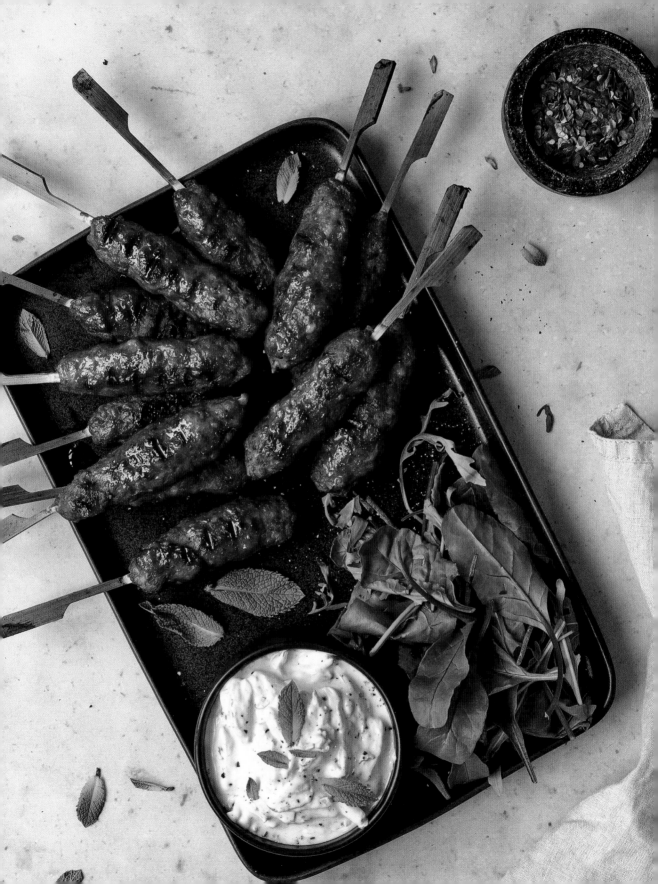

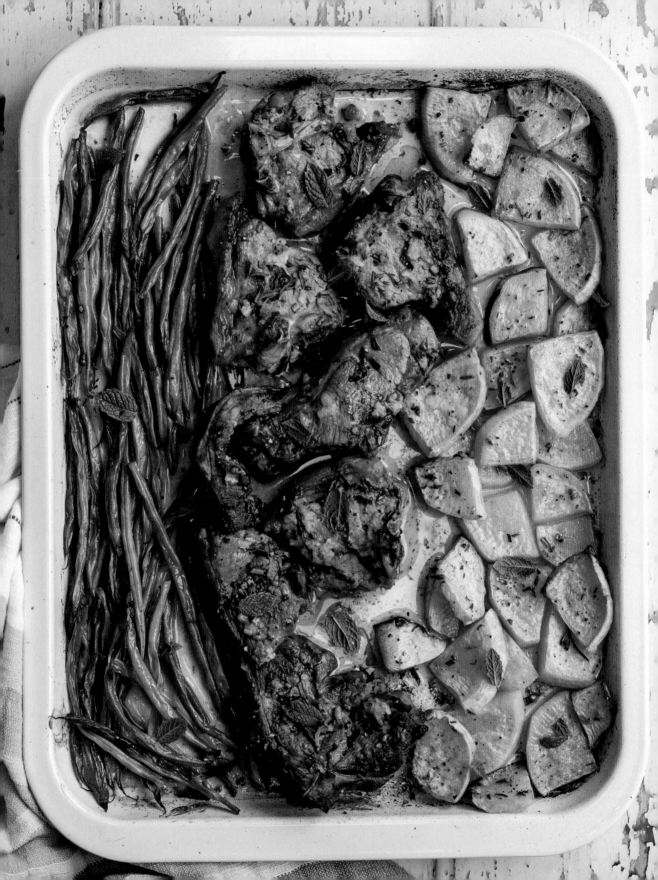

Sheet-Pan Herbed Lamb Chops

SERVINGS: 4
HANDS-ON TIME: 10 minutes
OVERALL TIME: 50 minutes

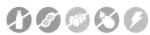

This tray bake is an easy keto dinner the whole family will love! You can add whatever non-starchy veggies you prefer. I like mine with rutabaga to swap for the commonly used potatoes, but you can use turnips, radishes, or sliced cauliflower.

4 tablespoons (60 ml) melted ghee,
  duck fat, olive oil, or avocado oil
1 clove garlic, minced
2 teaspoons (3 g/0.2 oz) chopped
  rosemary or ½ teaspoon dried
  rosemary
1 tablespoon (4 g/0.2 oz) chopped
  mint or 1 teaspoon dried mint
1 tablespoon (15 ml) lemon juice or
  apple cider vinegar
½ teaspoon salt, or to taste salt
Ground black pepper, to taste
1 medium (400 g/14.1 oz) rutabaga,
  peeled and cut into about ¼-inch
  (6 mm) slices
8 small (600 g/1.3 lb.) lamb chops
  (about 75 g/2.7 oz each)
7 ounces (200 g) green beans,
  trimmed

Preheat the oven to 400°F (200°C) forced fan or 425°F (220°C) conventional.

Mix the melted ghee, garlic, herbs, lemon juice, salt, and pepper in a bowl. Brush the rutabaga with about a third of the mixture, place in a baking tray, and bake in the oven for about 20 minutes, rotating the tray halfway through the cooking time.

Push the rutabaga to one side, add the lamb chops, brush with another third of the mixture, and bake for 10 minutes. Finally, add the green beans, drizzle with the remaining mixture, and bake for another 10 to 15 minutes.

Eat warm. Store in the fridge for up to 4 days.

TIP:

Need to drop the carb count? Swap the rutabaga for sliced turnips, halved radishes, or sliced daikon radish and only bake them for 10 minutes instead of 20 minutes.

NUTRITION FACTS PER SERVING (2 LAMB CHOPS + VEG):
Total carbs: 12.8 g / Fiber: 3.8 g / Net carbs: 9 g / Protein: 29.6 g / Fat: 36.9 g / Calories: 504 kcal
Macronutrient ratio: Calories from carbs (7%), protein (24%), fat (69%)

Chapter 8

Desserts

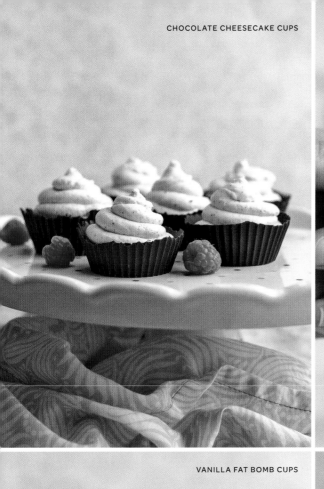

CHOCOLATE CHEESECAKE CUPS

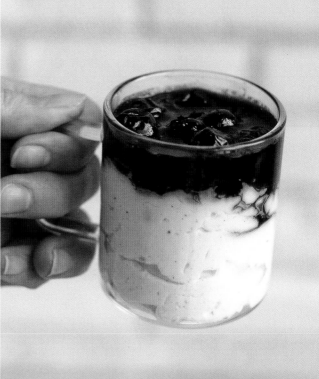

BLUEBERRY CHEESECAKE JARS

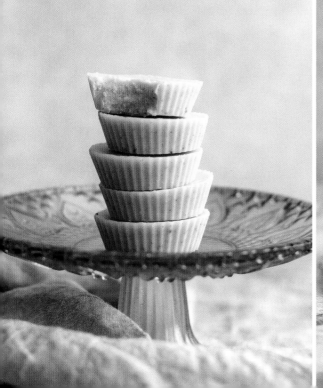

VANILLA FAT BOMB CUPS

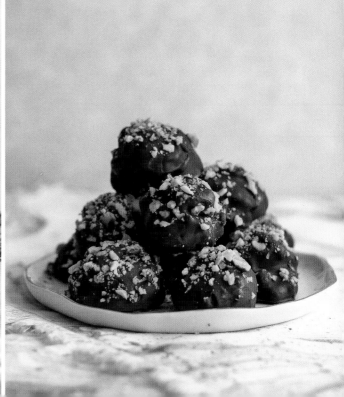

GIANT TRUFFLES TWO WAYS

Mochaccino Panna Cotta

Panna cotta is one of the easiest keto treats. It's ultra-low in carbs, high in fats, and has gut-healing gelatin protein. I make four servings for a healthy dessert-for-breakfast or six to eight small servings for an after-dinner treat.

13½ ounces (400 ml) heavy whipping cream or full-fat coconut milk

3 tablespoons (30 g/1.1 oz) powdered erythritol or Swerve

1 tablespoon (5 g/0.2 oz) cacao powder or Dutch-process cocoa powder

2 teaspoons (8 g/0.3 oz) instant coffee powder

1 teaspoon sugar-free vanilla extract

2 teaspoons (4 g/0.2 oz) gelatin powder

2 tablespoons (30 ml) filtered water

½ cup (120 ml) heavy whipping cream or coconut cream, whipped

Cinnamon, for dusting

Place the cream, erythritol, cacao powder, coffee powder, and vanilla in a saucepan. Heat over medium heat and stir until the sweetener has dissolved.

Sprinkle the gelatin powder over the 2 tablespoons (30 ml) cold water and set it aside to let it bloom. Once ready, add the bloomed gelatin to the hot cream mixture. Mix well until all the gelatin has dissolved.

Pour into four (4-ounce/120 ml) serving glasses and fill them about two-thirds full, leaving enough space for the whipped cream topping. Place in the fridge for 3 to 4 hours, or until set.

Add the whipped cream to the top of the panna cotta and dust with cinnamon. Store in the fridge for up to 4 days.

TIP:
Love tiramisu? Add a teaspoon of sugar-free rum extract to the panna cotta base and dust the cream with cacao powder.

NUTRITION FACTS PER SERVING:
Total carbs: 5 g / Fiber: 0.5 g / Net carbs: 4.5 g / Protein: 4.4 g / Fat: 50.1 g / Calories: 496 kcal
Macronutrient ratio: Calories from carbs (4%), protein (4%), fat (92%)

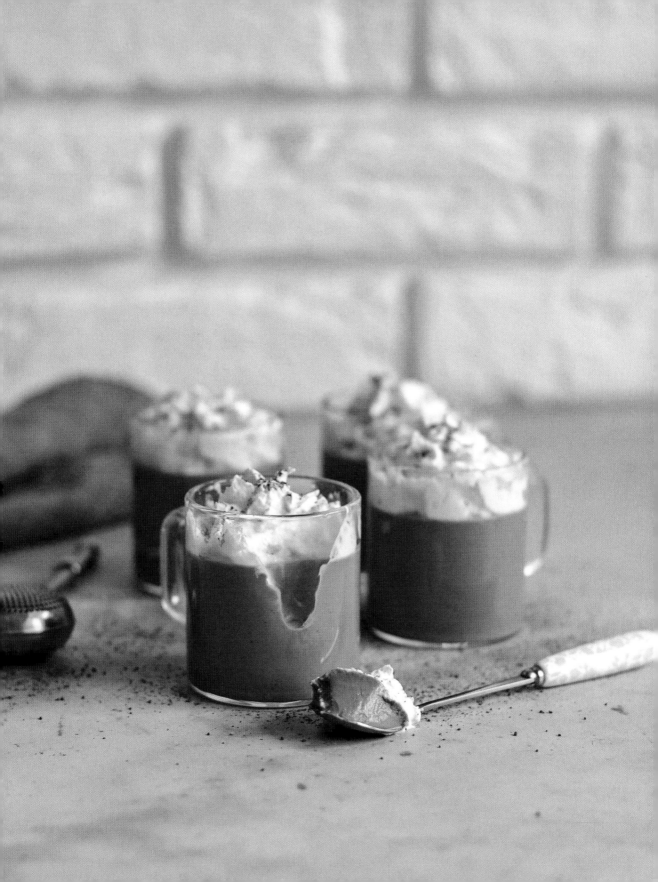

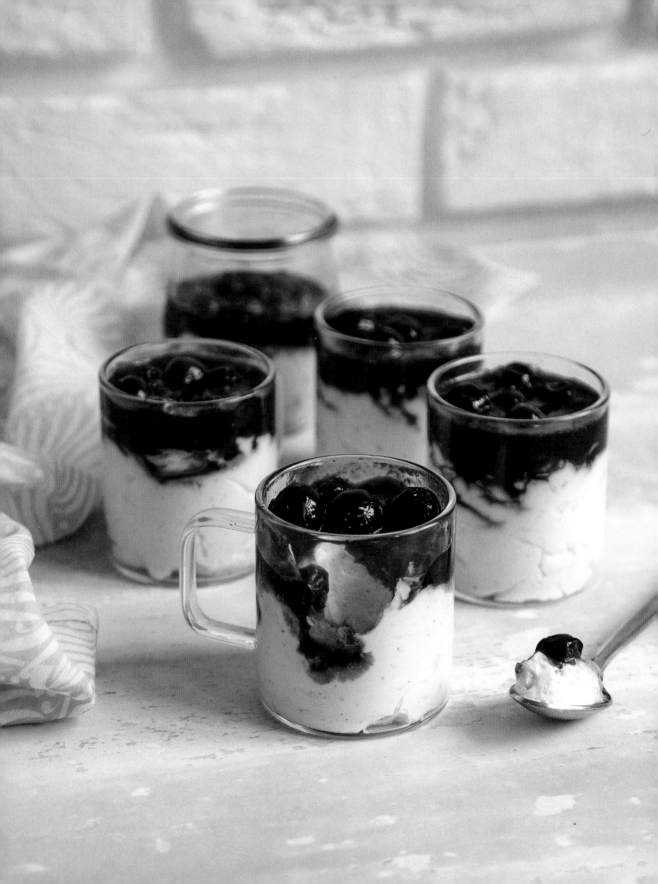

Blueberry Cheesecake Jars

SERVINGS: 5
HANDS-ON TIME: 15 minutes
OVERALL TIME: 20 minutes + chilling

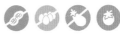

Creamy vanilla-lemon cheesecake topped with blueberry coulis, all in just fifteen minutes! To keep this recipe super simple, there is no baking involved and no crust needed!

BLUEBERRY TOPPING

1 cup (150 g/5.3 oz) wild fresh or frozen blueberries

1 tablespoon (15 ml) water

Optional: few drops of stevia, erythritol, or Swerve to taste

CHEESECAKE BASE

¾ cup (180 ml) heavy whipping cream

¾ cup (180 g/6.4 oz) full-fat cream cheese or mascarpone

¼ cup (58 g/2 oz) sour cream

¼ cup (40 g/1.4 oz) powdered erythritol or Swerve

1 teaspoon sugar-free vanilla extract

1 teaspoon fresh grated lemon zest

1 tablespoon (15 ml) fresh lemon juice

TO MAKE THE BLUEBERRY TOPPING: Place the blueberries and water in a saucepan. Gently heat over medium-low heat until the blueberries have softened. Optionally, add Stevia to taste. Remove from the heat and set aside to cool to room temperature. You can speed this up by placing the saucepan over a bowl with ice water.

TO MAKE THE CHEESECAKE BASE: Place all the cheesecake layer ingredients in a bowl. Using an electric mixer or a hand whisk, mix until smooth and creamy. Divide among five (4-ounce/120 ml) serving glasses and top with the blueberry sauce. You can serve these right away, but they are best chilled for at least 2 hours. Keep refrigerated for up to 4 days.

TIP:

You can make a quick keto-friendly crust by mixing ½ cup (50 g/1.8 oz) almond flour, ⅓ cup (25 g/0.9 oz) shredded coconut, ½ teaspoon cinnamon, pinch of salt, 1½ tablespoons (23 g/0.8 oz) unsalted butter or coconut oil, and optionally 1 tablespoon (10 g/0.4 oz) powdered erythritol or Swerve. Simply use as a no-bake base for the cheesecake jars.

NUTRITION FACTS PER SERVING:
TOTAL CARBS: 7 g / Fiber: 0.9 g / Net carbs: 6.1 g / Protein: 3.9 g / Fat: 26.2 g / Calories: 265 kcal
MACRONUTRIENT RATIO: Calories from carbs (9%), protein (6%), fat (85%)

Lemon Cake for Two

SERVINGS: 2
HANDS-ON TIME: 5 minutes
OVERALL TIME: 25 minutes

Sometimes the craving for a nice slice of cake will not go away. But if you cook just for yourself, making an entire cake seems like overkill. This keto-friendly treat only makes two generous servings and is perfect for portion control.

⅓ cup (33 g/1.2 oz) almond flour
¼ cup (50 g/1.8 oz) granulated erythritol or Swerve
1 teaspoon gluten-free baking powder
Optional: 1 teaspoon poppy seeds
1 large egg
2 tablespoons (30 ml) melted butter or coconut oil
1 teaspoon fresh lemon zest
1 tablespoon (15 ml) fresh lemon juice
2 tablespoons (30 ml) heavy whipping cream or coconut cream
¼ teaspoon sugar-free vanilla extract
Optional: mascarpone, crème fraîche, whipped cream, or coconut cream

Preheat the oven to 265°F (130°C) forced fan or 300°F (150°C) conventional. Place a small ovenproof saucepan filled with water in the oven. This will help the cake stay fluffy and prevent drying.

In a small bowl, combine the almond flour, erythritol, baking powder, and optionally poppy seeds. In another bowl, whisk the egg, butter, lemon zest, lemon juice, cream, and vanilla. Add the dry ingredients to the bowl and mix until well combined.

Divide the batter between two ramekins, 8 to 12 ounces (240 ml to 360 ml) each. Place in the oven and bake for about 20 minutes, or until set and lightly golden on top. Store at room temperature for 1 day or in the fridge for up to 5 days. Optionally, serve with mascarpone, crème fraîche, whipped cream, or coconut cream.

TIP:
For a quick dessert, microwave the cakes on high, one at a time, for about 90 seconds, checking halfway through the cooking time.

NUTRITION FACTS PER SERVING (1 CAKE):
Total carbs: 6 g / Fiber: 1.7 g / Net carbs: 4.3 g / Protein: 7.1 g / Fat: 28.4 g / Calories: 301 kcal
Macronutrient ratio: Calories from carbs (6%), protein (10%), fat (84%)

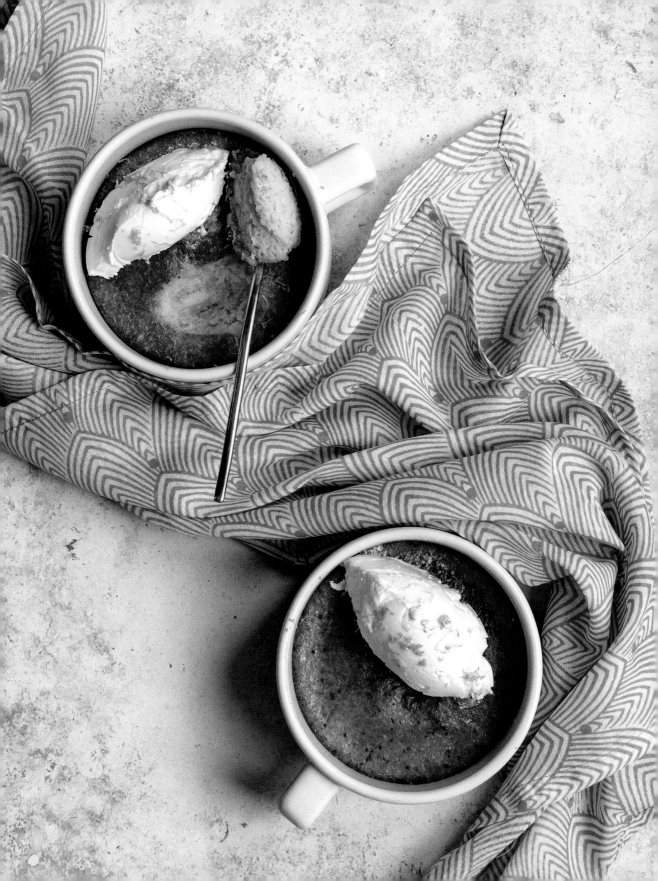

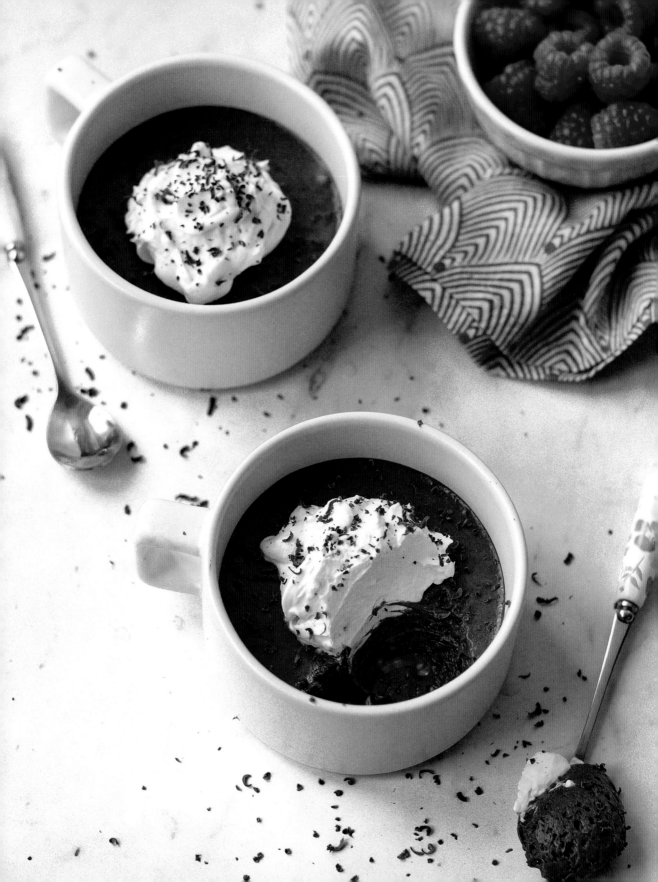

Dark Chocolate Mousse

SERVINGS: 4
HANDS-ON TIME: 15 minutes
OVERALL TIME: 15 minutes + chilling

This is my healthy low-carb take on a classic chocolate mousse recipe. For light, airy, and silky smooth texture, I followed the traditional approach of making chocolate mousse with fluffy egg whites, creamy dark chocolate, and butter. For an extra airy effect, you can fold in some whipped cream with the egg whites.

6 large squares (60 g/2.1 oz) unsweetened dark chocolate (100% cacao)

6 tablespoons (85 g/3 oz) unsalted butter

Pinch of salt

3 large eggs, separated

2 tablespoons (30 ml) filtered water

⅓ cup (67 g/2.4 oz) granulated erythritol or Swerve

1 teaspoon sugar-free vanilla extract

¼ teaspoon cream of tartar or ½ teaspoon fresh lemon juice

Optional: whipped cream (unsweetened or sweetened with a few drops of stevia or powdered sweetener), grated dark chocolate, and berries of choice

NOTE:
Worried about using raw eggs? Check out our tips for pasteurizing eggs on page 16.

Melt the dark chocolate in a double boiler, or use a heatproof bowl placed over a small saucepan filled with 1 cup (240 ml) of water and placed over medium heat. Remove from the heat and add the butter and salt. Stir to combine and let cool slightly. Alternatively, use a microwave and melt in short 10-to-15 second bursts until melted, stirring in between.

Separate the eggs in two bowls. Add the water, sweetener, and vanilla to the bowl with the egg yolks. Place the bowl over the saucepan of boiling water, and whisk until thickened, hot to the touch, and pale in color. Remove from the heat and set aside. In the second bowl, whisk the egg whites with the cream of tartar until they create soft peaks.

Drizzle the warm melted chocolate into the warm egg yolk mixture and beat until combined. Add about a third of the egg whites and beat in. Finally, use a rubber spatula to slowly fold in the remaining egg whites without deflating the mixture too much.

Divide among four ramekins or glasses (at least 4-ounce/120 ml each) and place in the fridge to set for at least 2 hours or overnight. Optionally, add a dollop of whipped cream, grated dark chocolate, and/or fresh berries on top. Store in the fridge for up to 4 days.

TIPS:
• You can keep your chocolate mousse super simple by only using 85% dark chocolate, butter, and eggs. Sweetener, vanilla, and cream of tartar can be omitted.
• For very smooth results, swap the erythritol for allulose. The carb count is the same as for erythritol, and it's as sweet as sugar. Unlike erythritol, it does not crystalize and is a great option in chilled desserts.

NUTRITION FACTS PER SERVING:
Total carbs: 3.3 g / Fiber: 0.9 g / Net carbs: 2.4 g / Protein: 7 g / Fat: 28.3 g / Calories: 278 kcal
Macronutrient ratio: Calories from carbs (3%), protein (10%), fat (87%)

Chocolate Cheesecake Cups

SERVINGS: 6
HANDS-ON TIME: 10 minutes
OVERALL TIME: 20 minutes

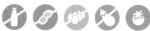

These simple keto fat bombs are so versatile and work with any cream, coconut cream, or buttercream filling. Feel free to add a pinch of cinnamon or a dash of any sugar-free extract. These cups are quite generous, and you can make up to twelve smaller servings if you prefer bite-size treats.

4 ounces (115 g) 90% dark chocolate

1 tablespoon (15 ml) virgin coconut oil or cacao butter

10.6 ounces (300 g) mascarpone, or ¾ cup (180 g/6.4 oz) cream cheese plus ½ cup (120 ml) heavy whipping cream

¼ cup (40 g/1.4 oz) powdered erythritol or Swerve

1 teaspoon sugar-free vanilla extract

1 teaspoon fresh lemon zest

Melt the dark chocolate and coconut oil in a double boiler, or use a heatproof bowl placed over a small saucepan filled with 1 cup (240 ml) of water and placed over medium heat. Let it cool to room temperature. Alternatively, use a microwave and melt in short 10-to-15 second bursts, stirring in between.

In a bowl, beat the mascarpone, erythritol, vanilla, and lemon zest. Place in the fridge and refrigerate until the chocolate cups are ready.

Place 6 medium silicone muffin cups in the freezer. Working one at a time, pour 1 tablespoon (15 ml) of the chocolate mixture inside the cups and swirl around. Place back in the freezer to solidify. Pour about ½ a tablespoon (7 ml) of the melted chocolate in each cup and swirl around to create a rim (each cup should be about 22 g/0.8 oz). Keep in the fridge until ready to fill. Remove from the fridge and gently release the cups.

Transfer the cooled cheesecake mixture to a piping bag fitted with a medium or large star tip. Pipe the cheesecake mixture inside each of the 6 cups (about 57 g/2 oz of filling per cup). Store in the fridge in a sealed jar for up to 5 days.

TIPS:

• Are you dairy-free? Instead of mascarpone cheese, use coconut cream or thick coconut yogurt.

• Instead of 90% dark chocolate, you can use any chocolate with at least 85% cacao solids, or sugar-free chocolate. You can even make your own. Check out my recipe at ketodietapp.com/blog.

• Love buttercream? Instead of the cheesecake filling, you can swap for chocolate buttercream filing from the Yellow Butter Cake Cupcakes (page 164).

NUTRITION FACTS PER SERVING (1 CUP):
Total carbs: 5.1 g / Fiber: 1.3 g / Net carbs: 3.8 g / Protein: 4.8 g / Fat: 30.7 g / Calories: 307 kcal
Macronutrient ratio: Calories from carbs (5%), protein (6%), fat (89%)

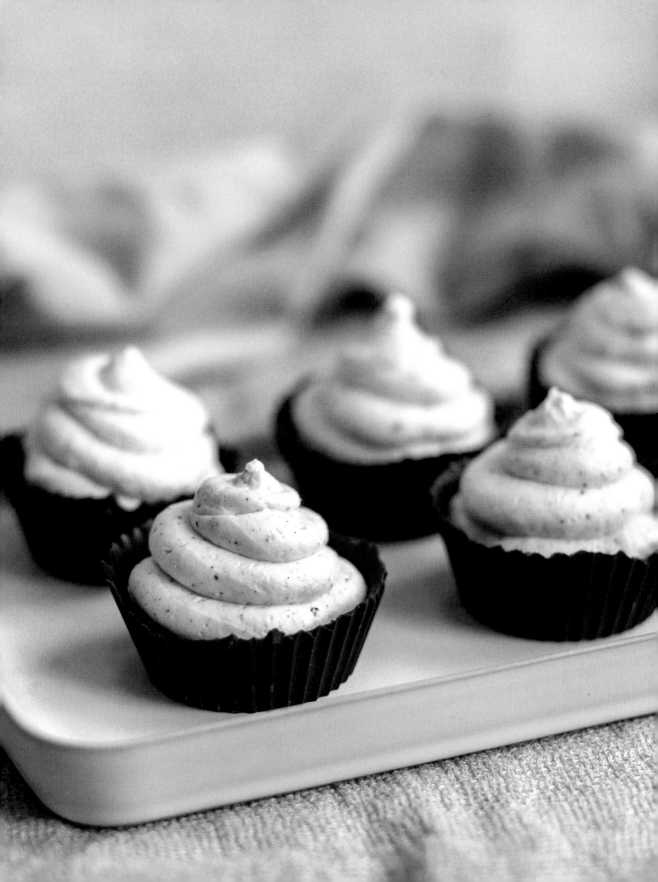

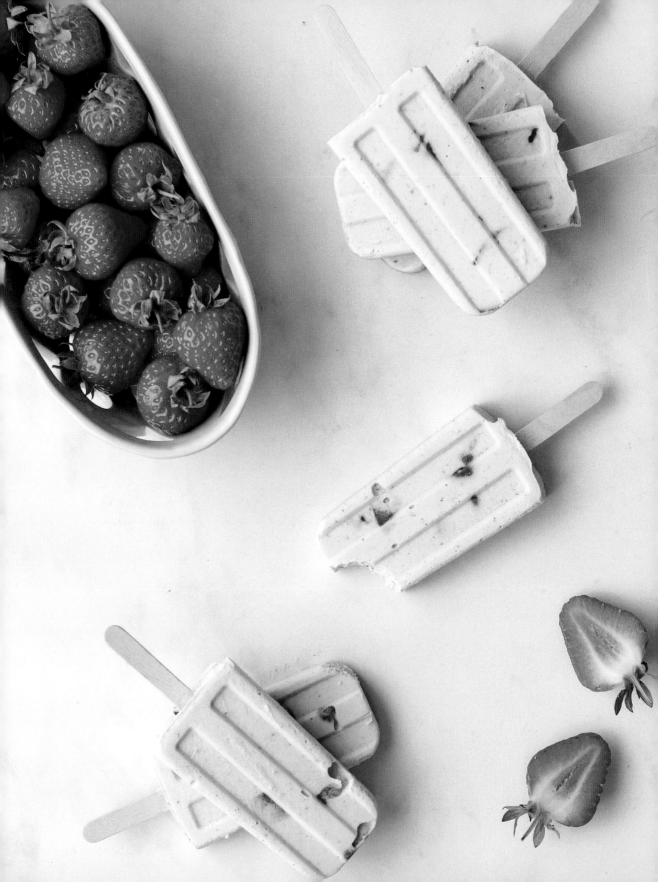

3-Ingredient Strawberry Popsicles

SERVINGS: 8
HANDS-ON TIME: 10 minutes
OVERALL TIME: 3 to 4 hours freezing

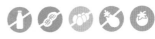

I love the simplicity of these berry popsicles! They are sweetener-free, but you can add a few tablespoons of powdered low-carb sweetener or a few drops of stevia. Feel free to swap for other berries, too.

10.6 ounces (300 g) fresh or frozen and thawed strawberries

10.6 ounces (300 g) mascarpone or heavy whipping cream

1 tablespoon (15 ml) sugar-free vanilla extract

OPTIONAL ADD-INS

¼ cup (40 g/1.4 oz) powdered erythritol or Swerve, or stevia drops to taste

1 tablespoon (15 ml) MCT oil to help reduce iciness

3½ ounces (100 g) melted dark chocolate for coating (at least 85% cacao or sugar-free)

Shredded coconut, slivered almonds, or chopped pecans for topping

Place the strawberries, mascarpone, and vanilla in a blender and process until smooth and creamy. Optionally, blend with the sweetener and MCT oil. You optionally can reserve a few chopped strawberries and add them to the mixture after blending. Pour into regular 3-ounce (80 ml) popsicle molds, or in more small popsicle molds.

Freeze for 3 to 4 hours, or until fully set. To release the popsicles from the molds, briefly dip the popsicle molds in a pot of hot water. If you're using chocolate coating, make sure the melted chocolate has cooled to room temperature before dipping the frozen popsicles into it. If you're adding coconut or other nut toppings, sprinkle them on top before the coating has set and place the popsicles back in the freezer until fully set. Store in a plastic bag in the freezer for up to 3 months.

TIP:

Mascarpone is high in fat and will make the popsicles creamier, but you can always sub for heavy whipping cream or with cream combined with cream cheese (for a cheesecake-like flavor). If you are dairy-free, use coconut cream or coconut yogurt instead.

NUTRITION FACTS PER SERVING (1 POPSICLE):
Total carbs: 3.6 g /Fiber: 0.8 g /Net carbs: 2.8 g / Protein: 2.4 g /Fat: 13.3 g /Calories: 147 kcal
Macronutrient ratio: Calories from carbs (8%), protein (7%), fat (85%)

Double Chocolate Chip Cookies

SERVINGS: 8
HANDS-ON TIME: 10 minutes
OVERALL TIME: 2 hours

These cookies were part of a trio of recipes I was working on to finalize my ultimate guide to keto cookies. It took a lot of fine-tuning to find that one perfect cookie recipe. The hardest part was to avoid xanthan gum, a common ingredient in gluten-free baking that seemed essential for the texture because it prevents crumbliness. The problem is that it is not always well tolerated and may cause tummy issues. I found that the right combination of keto ingredients and the addition of psyllium really helps avoid that unwanted extra-crumbly texture.

¾ cup (75 g/2.7 oz) almond flour

1½ tablespoons (12 g/0.4 oz) coconut flour

⅓ cup (28 g/1 oz) cacao powder or Dutch-process cocoa powder

1 tablespoon (8 g/0.3 oz) powdered psyllium husks

1 teaspoon gluten-free baking powder, or ¼ teaspoon of baking soda plus ½ teaspoon cream of tartar

½ cup (113 g/4 oz) unsalted butter at room temperature

⅓ cup (67 g/2.4 oz) erythritol or Swerve

1 large egg

1 teaspoon sugar-free vanilla extract

½ cup (50 g/1.8 oz) pecans, chopped

⅓ cup (60 g/2.1 oz) dark chocolate chips or chopped dark chocolate (any 85% to 100% chocolate will work)

Flaked sea salt, to taste

Place the almond flour, coconut flour, cacao powder, psyllium powder, and baking powder in a mixing bowl. Using an electric mixer, process until well combined.

In another bowl, using an electric mixer, cream the butter with the erythritol. Add the egg and vanilla and keep mixing until well combined. Add about a third of the dry mixture and mix well. Add the remaining two-thirds and mix until well combined.

Add the chopped nuts and chocolate chips, and fold in using a spatula. To make the cookies prettier, you can leave part of the chocolate and nuts for topping. Place in the fridge for 30 to 60 minutes. The mixture should be less sticky but not too solid to scoop.

When you're ready to make the cookies, preheat the oven to 320°F (160°C) forced fan or 355°F (180°C) conventional. Line a baking sheet with parchment paper.

Use a spoon or a cookie scoop to create eight equally sized mounds (about 58 g/2 oz each) and place them on the baking sheet. Make sure there is enough space as they will spread by ½ to 1 inch (1 to 2.5 cm). Using your hands, flatten the dough slightly. Bake for 10 to 12 minutes, checking halfway. If one side gets darker than the other, rotate the tray.

Remove the cookies from the oven and let them cool completely before moving the cookies off the tray. The cookies will be very fragile at first but will crisp up as they cool, within 1 to 2 hours. Store in a cookie jar for up to 1 week or freeze for up to 6 months.

NUTRITION FACTS PER SERVING (1 COOKIE):
Total carbs: 8 g / Fiber: 4.3 g / Net carbs: 3.7 g / Protein: 5.2 g / Fat: 26.4 g / Calories: 269 kcal
Macronutrient ratio: Calories from carbs (5%), protein (8%), fat (87%)

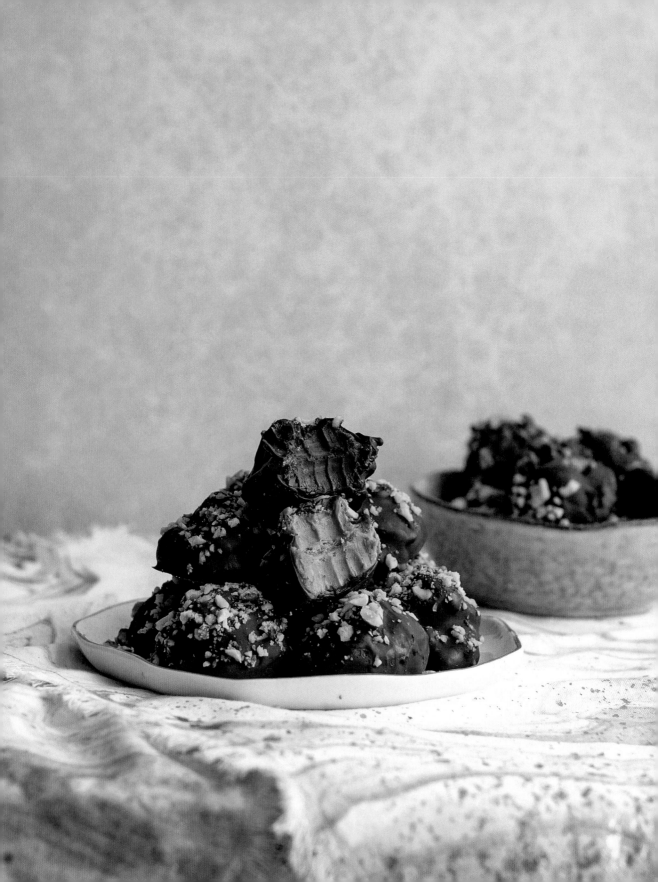

Giant Truffles Two Ways

SERVINGS: 6
HANDS-ON TIME: 15 minutes
OVERALL TIME: 1 hour

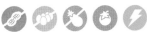

These easy truffles are everything you want in a healthy keto treat. They are rich and creamy with a smooth, nutty filling and a crunchy chocolate coating. I like my truffles big because they take less time to prepare and are more satisfying, but you can make up to twelve small truffles if you prefer them bite-size.

GIANT COOKIE DOUGH TRUFFLES

½ cup (125 g/4.4 oz) softened roasted almond butter

6 tablespoons (85 g/3 oz) unsalted butter, at room temperature

3 tablespoons (30 g/1.1 oz) powdered erythritol or Swerve

1 teaspoon fresh lemon zest

1½ teaspoons sugar-free vanilla extract

GIANT CHOCOLATE TRUFFLES

½ cup (125 g/4.4 oz) softened roasted almond butter

6 tablespoons (85 g/3 oz) unsalted butter, at room temperature

¼ cup (40 g/1.4 oz) powdered erythritol or Swerve

¼ cup (22 g/0.8 oz) cocoa powder or Dutch-process cocoa powder

¼–½ teaspoon ground cinnamon

Pinch of salt

COATING

½ bar (50 g/1.8 oz) 90% dark chocolate or dark chocolate with at least 85% cacao solids, or sugar-free chocolate

1 tablespoon (14 g/0.5 oz) cacao butter

2 tablespoons (14 g/0.5 oz) chopped pecans, shredded coconut, slivered almonds, or cacao nibs, for sprinkling

TO MAKE THE TRUFFLES: Place all the ingredients for the truffle filling in a bowl. Use an electric mixer to process until smooth and creamy. Place the mixture in the fridge for about 1 hour. Remove from the fridge and use a cookie scoop to make 6 large mounds (each about 41 g/1.5 oz for the cookie dough, and 45 g/1.5 oz for the chocolate). Place in the freezer for about 30 minutes. Don't worry if they are not perfectly round.

TO MAKE THE COATING: Melt the dark chocolate and cacao butter in a double boiler, or use a heatproof bowl placed over a small saucepan filled with 1 cup (240 ml) of water and placed over medium heat. Remove from the heat and let cool to room temperature before using for coating. Alternatively, use a microwave and melt in short 10-to-15 second bursts until melted, stirring in between.

Gently pierce each very cold truffle with a toothpick or a fork. Working one at a time, hold the truffle over the melted chocolate and spoon the chocolate over it to coat completely. Turn the toothpick as you work until the coating is solidified. Place the coated truffles on a parchment-lined tray and drizzle any remaining coating over them. Before they become completely solid, sprinkle with chopped nuts.

Refrigerate the coated truffles for at least 15 minutes to harden. Keep refrigerated for up to 1 week or freeze for up to 3 months.

TIPS:

• If you can tolerate peanuts, swap the almond butter for smooth or chunky roasted peanut butter. For nut-free truffles, use sunflower seed butter or coconut butter (aka coconut manna, *not* coconut oil or coconut cream).

• Cacao butter can be replaced with coconut oil. Keep in mind that coconut oil melts unless you keep it refrigerated.

NUTRITION FACTS PER SERVING (1 COOKIE DOUGH/CHOCOLATE TRUFFLE):
Total carbs: 6.2/8.4 g / Fiber: 2.9/4.3 g / Net carbs: 3.3/4.1 g / Protein: 5.5/6.2 g / Fat: 31.7/32.2 g / Calories: 316/322 kcal
Macronutrient ratio: Calories from carbs (4/5%), protein (7/8%), fat (89/87%)

Just-Like-Apple Crumble Coffee Cake

SERVINGS: 16
HANDS-ON TIME: 15 minutes
OVERALL TIME: 45 minutes

Apple pie has always been my favorite treat. The smell of cinnamon and baked apples in my mom's kitchen brings back so many great memories. I was surprised by how close zucchini tastes to apples when you bake it with cinnamon, sweetener, and some lemon juice. This cake tastes so good that none of my non-keto friends and family were able to tell the difference!

ZUCCHINI APPLE LAYER

3 medium (640 g/1.4 lb.) zucchini, peeled and core removed (440 g/15.5 oz edible parts)
2 tablespoons (30 ml) fresh lemon juice
¼ cup (40 g/1.4 oz) granulated erythritol, Swerve, or brown sugar substitute
1 teaspoon ground cinnamon

CAKE

2 cups (200 g/7.1 oz) almond flour
¼ cup (30 g/1.1 oz) coconut flour
1 tablespoon (8 g/0.3 oz) powdered psyllium husks
1 tablespoon (12 g/0.4 oz) gluten-free baking powder, or 1½ teaspoons cream of tartar plus ¾ teaspoon baking soda
¼ teaspoon salt
1½ teaspoons ground cinnamon, plus more for dusting
½ cup (43 g/1.5 oz) unsalted butter
¾ cup (150 g/5.3 oz) granulated erythritol, Swerve, or brown sugar substitute
4 large eggs
1 teaspoon sugar-free vanilla extract
½ cup (120 ml) unsweetened almond milk, at room temperature

CRUMBLE TOPPING

1½ cups (150 g/5.3 oz) almond flour
3 tablespoons (30 g/1.1 oz) granulated erythritol, Swerve, or brown sugar substitute
3 tablespoons (42 g/1.5 oz) unsalted butter, cut into pieces
1 teaspoon sugar-free vanilla extract or ground cinnamon

Whipped cream or full-fat yogurt, for serving

TO MAKE THE ZUCCHINI APPLE LAYER: Peel the zucchini, cut in half lengthwise, and scoop out the seeds using a melon baller or teaspoon. You can use the core for another recipe or discard. Chop into ¼-inch (6 mm)-thick slices. Place in a bowl and mix with the lemon juice. Set aside.

TO MAKE THE CAKE: Preheat the oven to 350°F (175°C) forced fan or 380°F (195°C) conventional. Line a cake pan with parchment paper; any pan close to 15 x 11 x 1 inch (39 x 29 x 2.5 cm) will be ideal.

In one bowl, mix all the dry ingredients for the cake. In another bowl, using an electric mixer, cream the butter with the erythritol. Add the eggs and vanilla and keep mixing until well combined. Add the almond milk and mix well. Add about a third of the dry mixture and combine well. Add the remaining two-thirds and mix until well combined.

Pour the cake batter into the lined cake pan. Top with the zucchini slices, sprinkle with the sweetener, and dust with the cinnamon. Place in the oven and bake for about 30 minutes.

TO MAKE THE CRUMBLE TOPPING: Place all the ingredients in a bowl and use your hand to combine well until you get a thick, sticky dough. After the cake has been baking for 30 minutes, crumble the dough on top of the cake and place back in the oven for another 10 minutes.

Remove from the oven and let the cake cool. Serve with whipped cream or full-fat yogurt. Store at room temperature for 1 day, in the fridge for up to 5 days, or slice and freeze for up to 3 months.

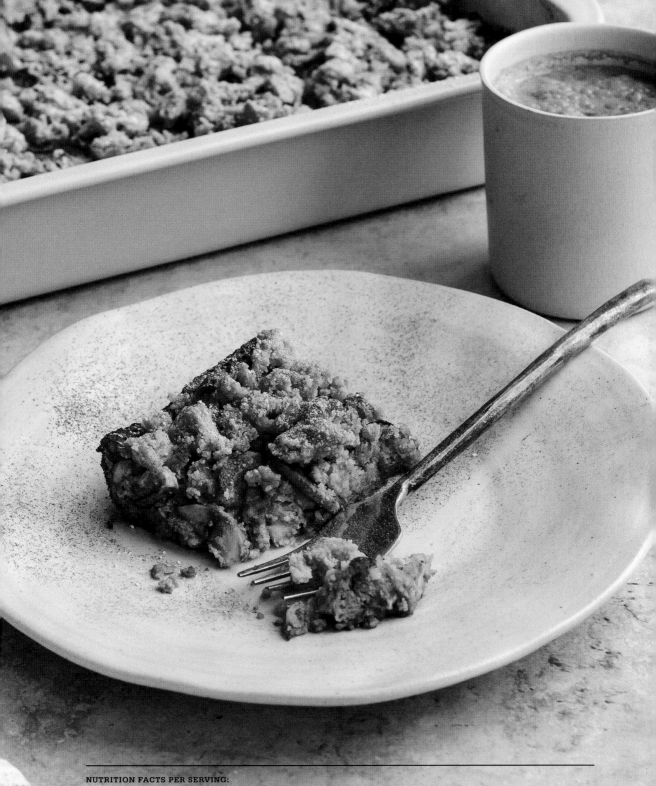

NUTRITION FACTS PER SERVING:
Total carbs: 7.3 g / Fiber: 3.3 g / Net carbs: 4 g / Protein: 7.1 g / Fat: 21.1 g / Calories: 236 kcal
Macronutrient ratio: Calories from carbs (7%), protein (12%), fat (81%)

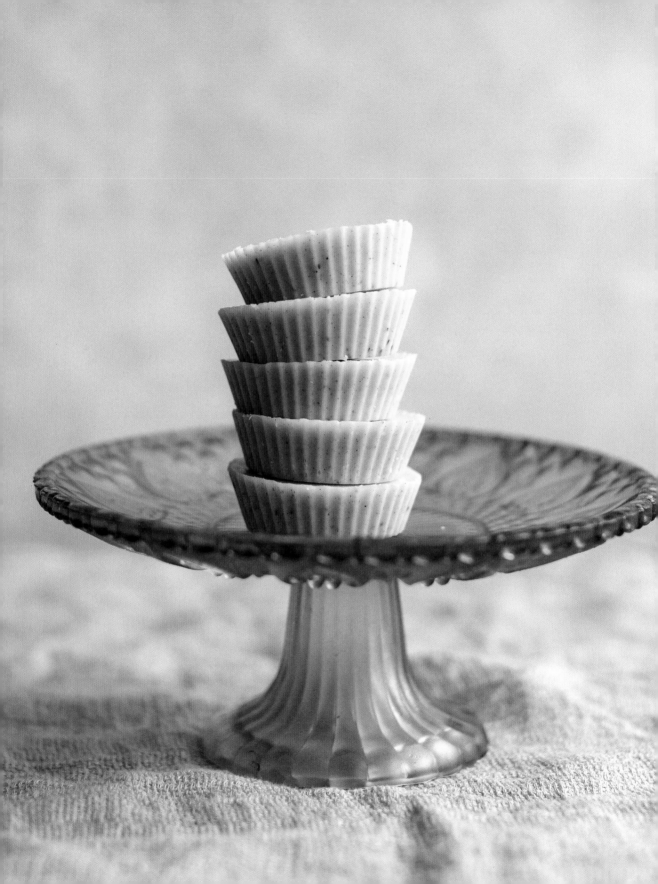

Vanilla Fat Bomb Cups

SERVINGS: 6
HANDS-ON TIME: 10 minutes
OVERALL TIME: 1 hour

These cups taste a bit like white chocolate. They are allergy-friendly and can even be made sweetener-free. Feel free to mix and match any of the suggested extras!

½ cup (125 g/4.4 oz) coconut butter (aka coconut manna, *not* coconut oil or coconut cream)

2 tablespoons (28 g/1 oz) cacao butter

½ teaspoon vanilla bean powder or 1 teaspoon sugar-free vanilla extract

2 tablespoons (20 g/0.8 oz) powdered erythritol or Swerve

Melt the coconut butter and cacao butter in a double boiler, or use a heatproof bowl placed over a small saucepan filled with 1 cup (240 ml) of water and placed over medium heat. Remove from the heat. Alternatively, use a microwave and melt in short 10-to-15 second bursts until melted, stirring in between.

Divide the mixture among six medium silicone muffin cups (about 2 tablespoons/30 ml each) and refrigerate for 30 to 45 minutes, until fully set. Keep refrigerated for up to 2 weeks or freeze for up to 6 months.

TIPS:

• Swap the coconut butter for any nut or seed butter. Blanched almond butter is a great alternative!

• Swap the cacao butter for virgin coconut oil.

• Add 1 to 2 tablespoons (7 to 14 g/0.3 to 0.6 oz) of collagen powder for extra protein and gut-healing gelatin.

• Swap the vanilla for cinnamon or lemon zest.

• Swap the erythritol for stevia drops (use to taste) or avoid sweetener altogether.

• Add chopped nuts or seeds, flaked toasted coconut, cacao nibs, chopped dark chocolate, or freeze-dried berries on top.

NUTRITION FACTS PER SERVING:
Total carbs: 4.6 g / Fiber: 3.1 g/ Net carbs: 1.5 g/ Protein: 1.3 g/ Fat: 16 g/ Calories: 159 kcal
Macronutrient ratio: Calories from carbs (4%), protein (3%), fat (93%)

Yellow Butter Cake Cupcakes

SERVINGS: 8
HANDS-ON TIME: 15 minutes
OVERALL TIME: 1 hour 30 minutes

These cupcakes are a healthier version of the popular yellow butter cake. It's a rich coffee cake that gets its beautifully yellow color from extra egg yolks. These cupcakes also freeze well, including the frosting!

CUPCAKES

1 cup (100 g/3.5 oz) almond flour

2½ tablespoons (20 g/0.7 oz) coconut flour

1 teaspoon gluten-free baking powder

6 tablespoons (85 g/3 oz) unsalted butter, at room temperature

⅓ cup (67 g/2.4 oz) granulated erythritol or Swerve

2 large eggs

2 egg yolks

2 teaspoons (10 ml) sugar-free vanilla extract

CHOCOLATE FROSTING

4.4 ounces (125 g) unsalted butter, at room temperature

¼ cup (22 g/0.8 oz) cacao powder or Dutch-process cocoa powder

¼ cup (40 g/1.4 oz) powdered erythritol or Swerve

¼ cup (60 ml) heavy whipping cream

1 teaspoon sugar-free vanilla extract

Preheat the oven to 320°F (160°C) forced fan or 355°F (180°C) conventional.

TO MAKE THE CUPCAKES: Place the almond flour, coconut flour, and baking powder in a bowl. Using an electric mixer, process until well combined.

In another bowl, using an electric mixer, cream the butter with the erythritol. Add the eggs, egg yolks, and vanilla and keep mixing until well combined. Add about a third of the dry mixture and mix well. Add the remaining two-thirds and mix until well combined.

Spoon the dough into eight lightly greased medium-size muffin paper cups (or silicone cups) placed in a muffin pan. Place in the oven and bake for 25 to 30 minutes. If one side starts to get darker, rotate the pan to ensure even baking. The cupcakes are done when a tooth-pick inserted into the middle comes out clean. Remove from the oven and let the cupcakes cool down completely before adding the frosting.

TO MAKE THE FROSTING: Place all the ingredients in a bowl and beat with an electric mixer until smooth and creamy. Spoon the frosting into a piping bag fitted with a medium or large star tip. Pipe the frosting onto the cupcakes (about 31 g/1.1 oz per cupcake).

Store in the fridge for up to 5 days or freeze for up to 3 months. The cupcakes taste best when they are left at room temperature for 15 to 20 minutes before serving.

TIP:

You can easily convert this recipe into a cake. To do that, simply pour the batter into a lined 8 x 8 inch (20 x 20 cm) baking pan. Bake until set in the middle and golden on top, about 30 minutes. Once the cake has cooled completely, spread the frosting on top.

NUTRITION FACTS PER SERVING (1 CUPCAKE):
Total carbs: 5.9 g / Fiber: 2.7 g / Net carbs: 3.2 g / Protein: 6.2 g / Fat: 33.7 g / Calories: 343 kcal
Macronutrient ratio: Calories from carbs (4%), protein (7%), fat (89%)

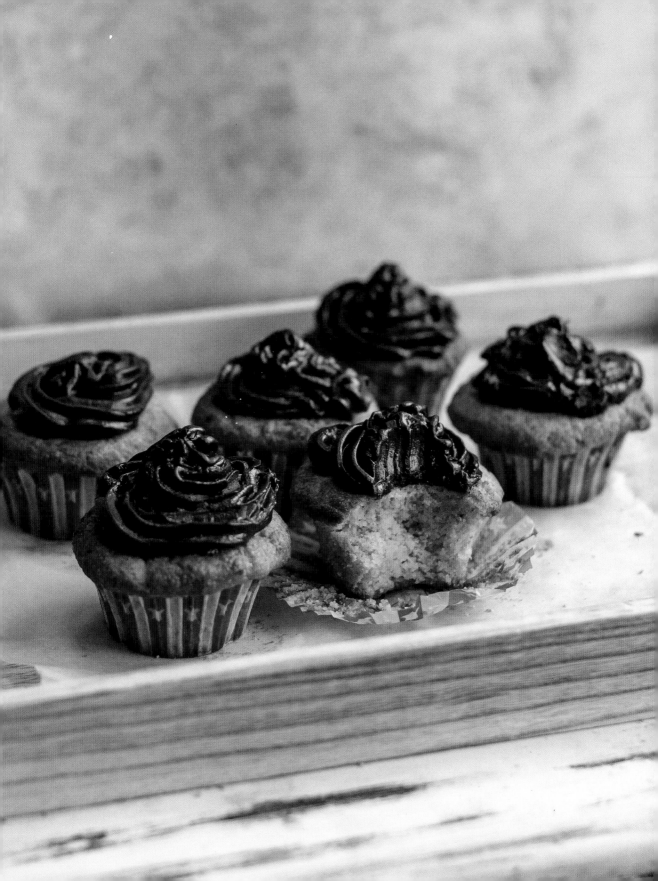

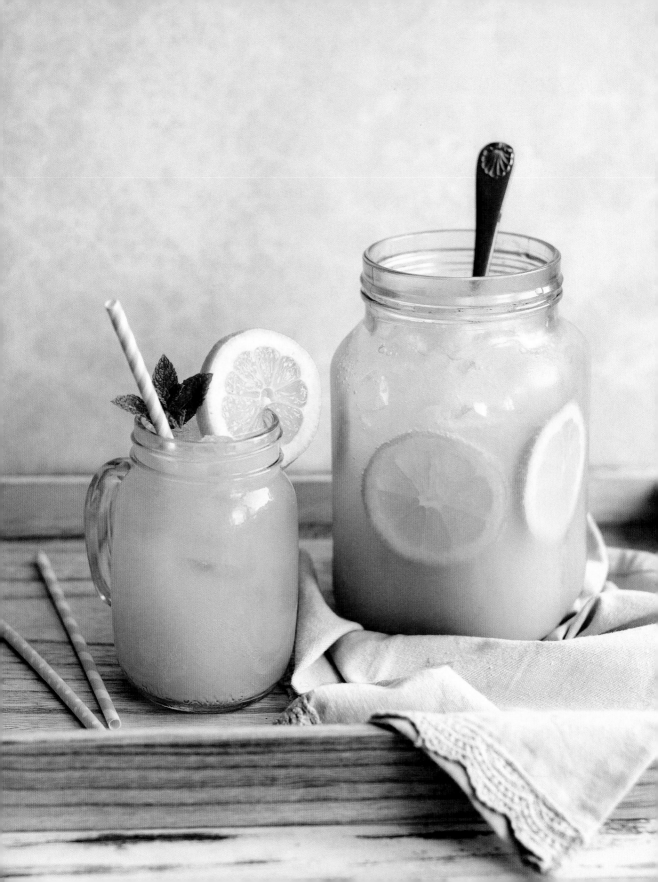

Ginger Lemonade

SERVINGS: 8
HANDS-ON TIME: 10 minutes
OVERALL TIME: 10 minutes

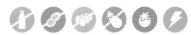

This lemonade tastes like lemon-flavored ginger beer. It's very refreshing and will satisfy your sweet tooth if you crave flavored beverages. If you want to drop the carbs by half, simply serve ¼ cup (60 ml) instead of the full serving and mix it with still or sparkling water to achieve the strength you like.

CONCENTRATE

1 piece (85 g/3 oz) fresh ginger, roughly chopped
2½ cups (600 ml) filtered water
1¼ cups (300 ml) fresh lemon or lime juice
½ cup (80 g/2.8 oz) powdered erythritol, Swerve, or brown sugar substitute

TO SERVE

1 cup (240 ml) still or sparkling water, or to taste
Lemon slices
Fresh mint
Ice

TO MAKE THE CONCENTRATE: Place the ginger in a blender together with 2½ cups (600 ml) filtered water. Process until all the ginger is blended. Pour through a fine-mesh sieve into a jug. Discard the leftover ginger trapped in the sieve.

To the jug, add the fresh lemon juice and powdered erythritol. Stir until the sweetener is completely dissolved. You can keep this concentrate in the fridge.

TO SERVE: Mix about ½ cup/120 ml concentrate with 1 cup sparkling water per serving. Add sliced lemon, mint, and ice to taste.

TIP:

It's easy to convert this recipe into a healthy electrolyte drink! Simply add 2 tablespoons plus 1½ teaspoons (16 g/0.5 oz) Natural Calm magnesium, ½ to ¾ teaspoon food-grade potassium chloride, and ¼ to ½ teaspoon sea salt. For best results, and to avoid stomach distress, always drink electrolyte drinks with meals, and do not exceed the recommended serving size. Sweeteners can be omitted; use them to taste. If you can't find potassium chloride, you can use ¾ to 1 teaspoon of Morton Lite Salt and skip the sea salt. It's ideal for after workouts or during the initial phase of the ketogenic diet when keto flu symptoms are more common.

NUTRITION FACTS PER SERVING (ABOUT ½ CUP/120 ML CONCENTRATE):
Total carbs: 5 g / Fiber: 0.3 g / Net carbs: 4.7 g / Protein: 0.3 g / Fat: 0.2 g / Calories: 19 kcal
Macronutrient ratio: Calories from carbs (87%), protein (6%), fat (7%)

References and Resources

ONLINE RESOURCES
KetoDiet Blog
www.ketodietapp.com/Blog

KetoDiet App
www.ketodietapp.com

How to Start Keto
www.ketodietapp.com/Blog/page/Start-Here

Keto Calculator (macronutrient calculator for low-carb diets)
www.ketodietapp.com/Blog/page/KetoDiet-Buddy

Facebook Support Group
www.facebook.com/groups/Ketodietplan/

BOOKS
The Beginner's Ketodiet Cookbook
Martina Slajerova

The Keto All Day Cookbook
Martina Slajerova

Keto Slow Cooker & One-Pot Meals
Martina Slajerova

The KetoDiet Cookbook
Martina Slajerova

Quick Keto Meals in 30 Minutes or Less
Martina Slajerova

Super Low-Carb Snacks
Martina Slaverova, Dana Carpendar, Landria Voigt

Sweet and Savory Fat Bombs
Martina Slajerova